Get Fit Without the Workout Program

The Lazy Girl's Guide

Eddie Bates

Disclaimer

Table of Contents

Overview

Welcome to "Get Fit Without the Workout Program: The Lazy Girl's Guide" to losing weight. This book is for you if you're sick of putting in countless hours at the gym and following rigid diet plans in an attempt to become a better, happier version of yourself.

Let's be honest, the conventional weight-loss method can be incredibly draining, time-consuming, and demoralizing. The temptation to work out for hours on end and closely monitor every bite you take can make it seem like an endless struggle that will never end, leaving you feeling defeated before you've ever started.

What if I told you that there's an alternative that might be just what you need? A method that doesn't call for you to give up all of your free time, give up your favorite meals or overnight become an exercise enthusiast. The purpose of this book is to demonstrate to you that you can reach your weight loss objectives without resorting to a conventional exercise regimen.

You'll find helpful advice, tactics, and insights in the pages that follow, all catered especially to the "lazy girl" in all of us. We'll look at simple yet powerful strategies to modify your lifestyle in a way that won't require drastic means or unattainable goals.

You'll see at the end of this book that there's no need to waste time on fads or unsustainable techniques that don't work. You'll discover that getting in shape and living a better life are achievable goals that don't have to seem laborious.

Therefore, there's no reason to let the conventional weight-loss strategy continue to dishearten and intimidate you. Say goodbye to guilt and taxing exercises, and welcome to a more straightforward and pleasurable path to better health. You won't regret it if you come along on this adventure to learn how to get healthy without following a workout regimen.

Chapter 1

Comprehending Loss of Weight Without Exercise

- **Dispelling myths and illusions**

There are many myths and misconceptions about weight reduction, which can cause confusion and frustration for those who are trying to reach their objectives. By confronting these misconceptions head-on, we can provide people with factual knowledge and pave the way for effective weight control.

The idea that exercise is the main factor in weight loss is a common misconception. Although exercise is undoubtedly important for overall health and can increase calorie expenditure, evidence indicates that dietary considerations are more important for initial weight loss. This fallacy can have its roots in the notion that exercising is the best way to burn calories and establish a calorie deficit. However, research indicates that consuming excess calories is far easier than burning them off with exercise alone. For instance, burning more calories in a single high-calorie meal than in a normal exercise session is quite possible. By breaking this myth, people can refocus on dietary changes that are more likely to help them reach their weight-loss goals.

The idea that some meals or minerals are intrinsically "bad" or "good" for weight loss is another widespread misconception. This binary approach to thinking can result in disordered behaviors or restrictive eating patterns because it oversimplifies the complicated relationship between nutrition and weight control. In actuality, weight gain or loss cannot be attributed to a single food or vitamin. Instead, weight status is determined by the overall balance between calories spent and calories consumed. Any item may be included in a balanced diet, and the key to enjoying a range of foods while still reaching weight loss objectives is moderation. People can embrace a more adaptable and sustainable eating style that prioritizes diversity, moderation, and balance by dispelling this myth.

Furthermore, there is a widespread perception that losing weight quickly is always desired and a sign of success. Fad diets and weight-loss plans that promise rapid results through severe calorie restriction or other extreme dietary restrictions contribute to the perpetuation of this fallacy. Rapid weight reduction, however, is frequently unsustainable and can have detrimental effects on one's health, such as muscle loss, nutrient shortages, and metabolic slowing, as evidenced by the study. Moreover, once regular eating patterns are restored, the weight lost during rapid weight loss is frequently gained back, creating a vicious cycle of yo-yo dieting and unhappiness. By busting this misconception, people can take a more measured and long-term approach to weight loss that puts long-term health and well-being ahead of immediate outcomes.

The idea that a person's ability to lose weight is determined by their genetics or specific body type is another common myth. Genetics can affect body composition, hunger hormones, metabolism, and other aspects of weight control, but it does not dictate a person's fate in this regard. Studies have demonstrated the importance of lifestyle factors in influencing weight status and overall health outcomes. These factors include nutrition, physical activity, sleep patterns, and stress management. Regardless of their genetic predispositions, people can take proactive steps towards achieving their weight loss goals by concentrating on elements within their control.

There's also a fallacy that says you have to follow a rigorous diet or food plan to lose weight. Although some people find structure and rules beneficial, strict diets sometimes result in feelings of shame, deprivation, and failure. Rather, concentrating on nutrient-dense, complete meals through flexible eating patterns can support a more pleasurable and long-lasting approach to weight loss. People can adopt a more flexible and intuitive eating style that promotes long-term success, enjoyment, and satisfaction by dispelling this fallacy.

Dispelling rumors and false beliefs is crucial to arming people with factual knowledge and assisting them in managing their weight. People can build enduring habits that promote their long-term health and well-being and gain a more nuanced view of weight reduction by dispelling popular misunderstandings about exercise, food choices, quick weight loss, heredity, and dietary rigidity.

Let's now examine more closely the doable methods for losing weight without the need for exercise, giving you the ability to take charge of your health and experience long-term achievement.

- ## The Science of Losing Weight

Creating techniques that work and support long-term success requires an understanding of weight loss's scientific underpinnings. Fundamentally, weight reduction is dictated by the energy balance principle, which says that changes in weight happen when the amounts of calories consumed and spent are different. This idea underpins almost all weight loss strategies and emphasizes how crucial it is to create a calorie deficit in order to promote fat loss.

→ **Intake and Extraction of Calories: The Energy Equilibrium Formula**

The energy balance equation provides a straightforward yet effective framework for comprehending changes in weight. According to this theory, weight gain results from the body storing extra energy as fat when calorie intake (calories in) exceeds calories expenditure (calories out). Weight loss, on the other hand, occurs when the body uses more calories from fat reserves to meet its energy needs than from calories consumed.

➔ Elements Affecting Energy Spending

Different energy expenditure components add to the body's total calorie burn. For most people, the largest portion of their overall energy expenditure is their basal metabolic rate (BMR), which represents the energy used at rest to sustain essential physiological functions including breathing, circulation, and cellular metabolism. BMR is influenced by a number of variables, including genetics, age, gender, and body composition; greater metabolic rates are generally linked to lean muscle mass.

Physical activity is a significant factor in determining total energy expenditure, in addition to BMR. This includes both non-exercise activities like walking, standing, and fidgeting as well as scheduled exercise activities like weightlifting, cycling, and running. Non-exercise activity thermogenesis (NEAT) is the term for even seemingly insignificant daily activities that can have a major impact on energy expenditure and aid in weight loss attempts.

Lastly, the energy required for the digestion, absorption, and metabolism of food nutrients is known as the thermic effect of food (TEF). TEF plays a role in overall energy balance and can fluctuate based on the macronutrient composition of the food, even though it makes up a smaller part of total energy expenditure than BMR and physical activity.

→ **The Secret to Losing Weight: Establishing a Calorie Deficit**

Since energy balance is the foundation of weight loss, establishing a calorie deficit is necessary to promote fat loss. This can be accomplished by combining dietary changes with increased physical activity, as these two factors add to the total energy deficit needed to lose weight.

Mindful eating, portion management, and calorie monitoring are a few examples of dietary interventions that try to lower caloric consumption. People can lower their overall calorie intake while still getting the nutrients they need by emphasizing nutrient-dense, whole meals, and consuming fewer processed and high-calorie items. Making protein-rich diets a priority can also aid in maintaining lean muscle mass and promoting satiety during weight loss.

Increasing physical activity levels can supplement dietary changes to further improve the calorie deficit and encourage fat loss. To increase calorie expenditure and enhance general fitness, this can be achieved through a mix of strength training, aerobic activity, and regular mobility. Maintaining a long-term devotion to an active lifestyle requires including pleasurable and sustainable activities.

→ **Elements That Influence Weight Loss Success**

The effectiveness of weight loss programs can be influenced by individual differences in metabolism, behavior, and environmental factors, even though the energy balance equation offers a theoretical framework for weight loss. Age, gender, genetics, hormone imbalances, illnesses, drugs, and psychological factors are just a few of the variables that might influence how someone reacts to food and lifestyle changes.

Success in losing weight is also influenced by social support, environmental cues, stress levels, mindset, and adherence to dietary and activity recommendations. To improve the effectiveness of weight loss endeavors, it is beneficial to employ methods that address key aspects such as setting attainable goals, acquiring stress management techniques, enhancing the quality of sleep, and developing a healthy and positive connection with food and body image.

Knowing the science of weight reduction provides people with the information and resources they need to make wise food and lifestyle choices. Through acknowledging the significance of energy equilibrium, maximizing energy intake and utilization, and tackling specific elements impacting weight reduction outcomes, people can create tailored approaches to accomplish and sustain their weight reduction objectives. The following pages will discuss ways to implement these ideas to take charge of your health and succeed in the long run.

- **Advantages of Losing Weight Without Working Out**

Exercise is frequently cited as being essential to losing weight; however, there are several advantages to losing weight without depending on regimented exercise regimens. Making dietary and lifestyle changes can have a substantial positive impact on those who are trying to lose weight, from increased mobility to better metabolic health.

★ Enhanced Joint Health and Mobility

It may be difficult or even impossible for those with orthopedic constraints, chronic pain disorders, or mobility issues to participate in traditional exercise activities. People can lose weight without making their current physical restrictions worse by concentrating on dietary adjustments and lifestyle improvements like portion control, mindful eating, and increased daily exercise. This may result in improvements in mobility, joint health, and overall quality of life, enabling people to move more easily and take part in activities they enjoy pain-free.

★ Lower Chance of Injuries Associated with Exercise

Exercises that are high-impact or demanding might raise the risk of musculoskeletal injuries, especially for those who are obese or overweight. Through dietary modifications and low-impact physical activities like cycling, swimming, or walking, people can lose weight without increasing their risk of injury from exercise. By putting safety and sustainability first, this strategy reduces the possibility of setbacks and lets people advance at their own speed.

★ Improved Cardiovascular and Metabolic Health

Studies have demonstrated that dietary modifications, such as cutting calories, selecting nutrient-dense foods, and maximizing the composition of macronutrients, can result in improvements in metabolic health indices like blood pressure, cholesterol, and sugar levels. People can reduce their risk of contracting chronic illnesses, such as type 2 diabetes, cardiovascular disease, and metabolic syndrome, by losing weight through dietary changes. Furthermore, increases in cardiovascular function, such as better circulation, heart health, and overall cardiovascular fitness, might result from changes in metabolic health.

★ Enhanced Adaptability and Ecological Balance

Dietary interventions have two of the main benefits of weight loss without exercise: adaptability and durability. In contrast to regimented workout plans that could call for certain gear, dedication, or physical effort, dietary adjustments can be tailored to meet personal tastes, way of life, and cultural background. Because of this flexibility, people can select dietary strategies that suit their own requirements and interests, which makes it simpler to stick to a diet plan over the long run and see long-term benefits in terms of weight loss.

★ Emotional and psychological advantages

Losing weight without exercising has many positive effects on psychological and emotional well-being, in addition to physical health. Putting an emphasis on nutritional interventions can help people who struggle to find satisfaction in physical activity or who have negative associations with exercise feel less stressed, anxious, or self-conscious about following typical exercise regimens. People can improve their body image, develop a positive relationship with food, and improve their general mental health by making dietary and lifestyle adjustments a priority.

★ Adequate and Reasonable Access

For those with limited resources or budgetary constraints, dietary interventions and lifestyle modifications are an appealing alternative to formal exercise programs since they are frequently more accessible and affordable. Dietary changes can be made using easily accessible resources and require less financial commitment than other fitness options like personal training, gym memberships, or equipment, which can be expensive and time-consuming. This accessibility promotes health justice and inclusivity by guaranteeing that weight-reduction interventions are available to people from a variety of socioeconomic backgrounds.

Chapter 2

Techniques for Mindful Eating

- EatingTips for Portion Control

Mastering portion control is essential to achieving successful weight management. Portion management is knowing how much food to consume and adjusting it so that it meets our demands for nutrients and our desired weight reduction. People may take charge of their eating habits and succeed in their weight reduction efforts for a long time by adopting mindful eating techniques and putting into practice helpful portion management advice.

➤ **Comprehending Portion**

MeasurementsKnowing what a typical portion size is is one of the first steps in implementing portion control. Today's culture has warped portion proportions, with large servings becoming the norm in fast-food restaurants, packaged goods, and dining establishments. Portion distortion is a phenomenon that has the potential to cause overeating and eventually contribute to weight gain.By using common items and visual clues as reference points, one may better grasp portion proportions. A serving of grains, such as rice, pasta, or bread, should be around the size of a tennis ball, but a portion of protein, such as meat, fish, or chicken, should be approximately the size of a deck of cards. Fruits and vegetables can be measured with the palm of your hand or a baseball, but fats and oils should only be measured with the size of your thumb.

➢ Mindful Food Practices

Eating with awareness involves observing all of the senses—taste, texture, scent, and sight—of the meal. By adopting mindful eating practices, people can reduce thoughtless eating, increase their awareness of hunger and fullness signals, and enjoy eating without overindulging.Slowing down and taking the time to really enjoy each mouthful of food, allowing yourself to completely absorb its tastes and sensations, is one effective mindful eating strategy. This makes it possible for people to gauge when they are full and refrain from overindulging. Serving yourself smaller quantities at first and then reevaluating your state of hunger before determining whether to have more is another aspect of careful portioning.Reducing distractions at mealtime, such as TV viewing, social media browsing, or computer use, is another beneficial tactic. People who only concentrate on the process of eating are better able to pay attention to their bodies' signals of hunger and fullness, which results in higher pleasure with lower serving sizes.

➢ Useful Advice on Portion Control

Apart from mindful eating practices, there are other pragmatic guidelines and tactics that people may use to regulate portion sizes and oversee their caloric consumption:

- Use smaller bowls and plates: Studies have shown that when given bigger dishes and bowls, individuals prefer to eat more. By utilizing smaller dishware, people can easily cut down on portion sizes without feeling deprived.
- Measure and measure food: Accurately portioning meals may help people avoid overindulging. This can be done with measuring cups, spoons, or a food scale. This is particularly beneficial for items like nuts, seeds, and granola that are prone to overindulgence.
- Proportion meals and snacks: When portions are made ahead of time and placed in snack-sized bags or grab-and-go containers, they may help reduce thoughtless overindulgence in food. This facilitates monitoring calorie consumption throughout the day and helps to regulate portion sizes.
- Follow the half-plate rule: Put non-starchy veggies (such as broccoli, bell peppers, and leafy greens) on half of your plate, and then split the other half between healthy grains and lean protein. This well-rounded strategy guarantees that you consume enough nutrients while also managing portion sizes.
- Be aware of liquid calories: Beverages, particularly sugary and alcoholic drinks, may add a lot of calories to our diets. To help you manage your total calorie consumption, choose low-calorie drinks like water, herbal tea, or other teas.

- When eating out, remember to watch your portion sizes. Restaurants often give large amounts, which makes it simple to overindulge. Before beginning your dinner, think about ordering an appetizer or side dish to go with your main course, sharing an entrée with a dining partner, or requesting a to-go container to divide out leftovers.
- It's important to pay attention to your body's signals of hunger and fullness, and to eat only when you are really hungry. Even if there is food left on your plate, you should stop eating when you are full. Maintaining a healthy relationship with food and avoiding overeating require understanding and respecting your body's natural cues of hunger and fullness.
- Eat consciously when you snack. If you don't snack mindfully, it might lead to calorie overload. Consider whether you're really hungry or are simply looking for a diversion before blindly grabbing for food out of habit or boredom. Select filling, nutrient-dense snacks like Greek yogurt with berries, fresh fruit, or veggies with hummus. To avoid overindulging, divide food into little bags or containers.
- Watch out for portion distortion. When dining out or consuming packaged meals, pay attention to portion distortion. Because restaurant servings are often larger than typical serving sizes, consider splitting a meal with a dining partner or requesting a half piece. Use measuring cups or a food scale to precisely divide out portions while consuming packaged meals. Nutrition labels usually provide the appropriate serving size.

- Measure portions using visual clues: If measuring cups or food scales are not accessible, estimate portion proportions using visual cues. Grain portions should be the size of your fist, protein portions your palm, and fat portions your thumb. Regular practice with portion estimation can help you get a better grasp of the right serving sizes.
- Planning and preparing meals in advance may help people control portion sizes and choose healthier foods throughout the week. Make time every week to organize your meals, make a shopping list, and prepare your items ahead of time. To make it simpler to get a healthy lunch when you're on the move or short on time, portion dishes into individual containers or serving sizes.
- Instead of adopting an all-or-nothing or restricted approach to eating, try practicing moderation rather than deprivation. This will allow you to enjoy your favorite foods in moderation. Not eating what you want may make you feel deprived and overeat. Instead, focus on mindful eating and portion management, prioritizing nutrient-dense, whole foods for most meals, and occasionally enjoying modest quantities of decadent foods.

You can take control of your eating habits, limit your calorie intake, and reach your weight loss goals without feeling deprived or constrained by adopting these useful portion management ideas into your daily routine. Remember that portion management is about making educated decisions and consuming food in a balanced, thoughtful manner, rather than rigid restrictions or deprivation.

● **Choosing foods high in nutrients**

The significance of selecting nutrient-dense foods in the quest for lasting weight reduction and overall health cannot be overemphasized. Foods that are abundant in vital nutrients—like vitamins, minerals, fiber, and antioxidants—in relation to their calorie level are considered nutrient-dense. You can ensure that you're getting all the nutrients you need while also encouraging satiety, bolstering metabolic health, and supplying your body with the fuel it needs to function at its best by giving these meals top priority in your diet.

➢ Knowledge of Nutrient Density

The ratio of nutrients to calories in a particular food is referred to as nutritional density. Nutrient-dense foods have a high concentration of vital nutrients in relation to their calorie level, which makes them very advantageous for general health and well-being. Conversely, foods with low nutrient densities, including processed snacks, sugary drinks, and refined carbs, may have a high calorie count but little nutritional benefit.Foods high in nutrients may take many different forms, but they usually consist of a variety of fruits, vegetables, whole grains, lean meats, and healthy fats. These foods are abundant in vital nutrients, such as vitamins, minerals, antioxidants, phytochemicals, and fiber. These nutrients are important for a number of physiological processes, including energy metabolism, immunological response, and cell regeneration and repair.

> ➤ **Crucial Foods High in Nutrients You Should Eat**

- Fruits and vegetables: Packed with vitamins, minerals, antioxidants, and fiber, fruits and vegetables are nutritional powerhouses. To optimize nutritional intake, try to include a range of vibrant fruits and vegetables in your meals and snacks. Whenever feasible, go for whole, less processed foods; furthermore, choose a rainbow of colors to guarantee a wide variety of nutrients.
- Whole Grains: Whole grains are a beneficial source of fiber, vitamins, minerals, and antioxidants. Examples of whole grains are brown rice, quinoa, oats, barley, and whole wheat. Complete grains maintain their nutritional integrity and provide long-lasting energy and fullness, in contrast to refined grains, which have had their nutrient-rich bran and germ removed. When selecting bread, pasta, cereal, and other grain-based items, look for whole-grain selections.
- Lean Proteins: Lean proteins are necessary for immunological response, hormone synthesis, muscle development, and repair and may be found in chicken, fish, tofu, tempeh, lentils, and low-fat dairy products. For diversity and balance in your diet, choose lean meats, skinless chicken, and fatty fish that are high in omega-3 fatty acids. You may also include plant-based protein sources in your meals.

- Healthy Fats: Essential for hormone balance, nutritional absorption, and brain function, healthy fats may be found in avocados, nuts, seeds, olive oil, and fatty seafood. Include foods high in healthy fats in your meals and snacks to increase fullness and improve the taste and texture of your food. Because fats are high in calories and may cause overconsumption if ingested in large amounts, it is important to watch portion proportions.
- Dairy and Dairy Alternatives: Rich in calcium, vitamin D, protein, and other vital elements, dairy products and dairy substitutes include milk, yogurt, cheese, and fortified plant-based milks. When feasible, go for low-fat or fat-free selections; to reduce additional sugars, choose unsweetened kinds.

➤ **Useful Advice for Selecting Foods High in Nutrients**

- Read nutrition labels: To determine the nutritional content and make wise decisions, carefully read nutrition labels when choosing packaged goods. Seek out foods that are rich in fiber, vitamins, and minerals and low in harmful fats, salt, and added sugars.
- Shop the Grocery Store's Periphery: Fresh, complete foods, such as fruits, vegetables, dairy products, and whole grains, are usually found along the periphery of the grocery store. To increase your nutrient intake and reduce your exposure to processed foods, focus your purchasing efforts on the perimeter.

- Meal Preparation and Batch Cooking: Allocate a certain period each week for meal planning and preparation. Large amounts of nutrient-dense meals, such as soups, stews, cereals, and roasted vegetables, may be prepared in bulk and portioned out for weekly consumption. Maintaining a nutrient-dense diet and reducing impulsive food choices may both be facilitated by having wholesome meals and snacks on hand.
- Include Superfoods: These are foods high in nutrients, especially vitamins, minerals, antioxidants, and other health-promoting substances. Berries, leafy greens, nuts, seeds, fatty fish, and whole grains are a few examples of superfoods. To optimize these foods' health-promoting properties, include them often in your meals and snacks.
- Eat with awareness: To fully appreciate the tastes and textures of nutrient-dense meals, eat slowly and carefully while paying attention to your body's signals of hunger and fullness. During mealtimes, be attentive and involved, and steer clear of distractions like television or electronics. Overeating may be avoided, and a deeper appreciation for the nutritious properties of food can be fostered by eating thoughtfully. You may optimize your nutrition, support your weight reduction objectives, and improve your general health and well-being by giving nutrient-dense foods top priority in your diet and implementing helpful guidelines for selecting better food choices.

Snacking allows you to avoid overeating at mealtime, satiate your appetite between meals, and feed your body nutrient-dense foods. Your energy levels will remain consistent throughout the day, and you may support your weight reduction objectives by selecting snacks that are delicious, well-balanced, and full of vital nutrients. Consider any of these suggestions for healthy snacks:

Fresh produce

Fruits provide a delectable blend of sweetness, fiber, vitamins, and antioxidants, making them nature's ideal snack. For a quick and portable snack, choose whole, fresh fruits like apples, bananas, oranges, berries, grapes, and kiwis. For maximum satiety and blood sugar balance, pair fruit with a healthy fat or protein source, such as Greek yogurt or a handful of almonds.

Sticks of vegetables with hummus

Crunchy veggie sticks and creamy hummus combine to provide a filling and healthy snack. To obtain a range of tastes and textures, use vibrant veggies like cherry tomatoes, bell peppers, cucumbers, carrots, and celery. Hummus is a pleasant and full dip because it contains fiber, protein, and healthy fats.

Greek Yogurt Parfait

Greek yogurt is a nutritious snack option for increasing satiety and intestinal health since it's high in protein and probiotics. For extra texture and taste, layer Greek yogurt with sliced bananas, fresh berries, and a dusting of oats or almonds. A Greek yogurt parfait is a filling midday snack or a simple, quick breakfast choice.

Apple slices with nut butter

For a tasty and wholesome snack, spread cashew, peanut, or almond butter on apple slices. Apples bring natural sweetness and fiber, while nut butter offers protein and healthy fats. This easy-to-make snack combo gives you long-lasting energy and fullness while satiating your sweet needs.

Pineapple-infused cottage cheese

Cottage cheese is a low-fat, high-protein dairy alternative that pairs well with tart and sweet fruits, such as pineapple. For a cool and filling snack, try a dish of cottage cheese with slices of fresh pineapple on top. Fiber and protein work together to keep you feeling content and full in between meals.

Mix Trail

Mix together a mixture of nuts, seeds, dried fruits, and dark chocolate chips to make your own trail mix. Dried fruits provide natural sweetness and antioxidants, while nuts and seeds offer fiber, protein, and healthy fats. Chips made with dark chocolate provide a decadent taste and extra health advantages. Divide the trail mix into bite-sized portions for an effortless on-the-go snack.

Tomato and avocado on rice cakes

For a crisp and filling snack, top whole-grain rice cakes with sliced tomatoes and mashed avocado. Tomatoes provide taste and freshness, while avocados offer heart-healthy fats. For more spice, add a dash of sea salt and black pepper. When you're in the mood for something hearty and satisfying, this snack is ideal.

Hard-boiled eggs

Rich in protein and other minerals, hard-boiled eggs make a handy and portable snack. Make a large batch of hard-boiled eggs at the start of the week and store them in the refrigerator for a simple and quick snack. Savor them without any accompaniments, or add some salt and pepper for a kick of flavor.

Edamame

Edamame, or steamed soybeans, are a high-fiber, high-protein, and micronutrient snack alternative. Edamame may be eaten as a snack on its own or added to salads, stir-fries, or grain bowls to give texture and additional protein. For extra flavor, sprinkle it with a little sea salt or your preferred spice combination.

Pudding with Chia

Packed with fiber, protein, and omega-3 fatty acids, chia pudding is a filling and creamy snack alternative. Mix chia seeds with your preferred milk (almond, coconut, or dairy) and a little amount of sweetener (stevia, honey, or maple syrup). To add more taste and texture, sprinkle fresh fruit, nuts, or seeds on top after letting the mixture thicken in the fridge for a whole night.

Hummus and veggie wraps

Line a whole grain or whole wheat tortilla with hummus, then top with sliced carrot, bell pepper, cucumber, and lettuce. Tightly roll the wrap, then cut it into bite-sized pieces for a filling and convenient snack. This wrap with veggies and hummus is a delicious alternative for a quick lunch or on-the-go snack.

Chickpeas, Roasted

Roasted chickpeas are a tasty and crispy snack that's high in protein, fiber, and minerals. Just sprinkle your chosen spices (paprika, cumin, garlic powder, or chili powder) with olive oil and canned chickpeas, then roast in the oven until golden and crispy. Savor roasted chickpeas by themselves or as a crisp garnish for grain bowls, salads, and soups.

Tuna salad with whole-grain crackers

Serve store-bought or homemade tuna salad over whole-grain crackers for a filling and high-protein snack. Whole-grain crackers supply fiber and complex carbs, while tuna salad supplies protein and beneficial fats. For the healthiest choice, look for crackers made mostly of whole grains with little to no additional additives.

Bowl of Smoothies

To make a thick and creamy smoothie bowl, blend your preferred fruits, veggies, protein powder, and liquid. Transfer the smoothie into a bowl and garnish with a selection of wholesome ingredients, including granola, shredded coconut, almonds, and seeds. Smoothie bowls are a healthy and adaptable snack choice that work well for lunch, breakfast, or a midday energy boost.

Oven-cooked sweet potato fries

Cut sweet potatoes into thin strips, mix with your preferred spices (such as garlic powder, smoked paprika, and sea salt), and bake in the oven until crispy and golden. Sweet potato fries that are baked are a tasty and healthy substitute for regular French fries since they are high in antioxidants, vitamins, and fiber. Enjoy them on their own, or add a little flavor by dipping them in guacamole or hummus.

Seaweed Appetizers

Seaweed snacks are a salty and crunchy food that is high in antioxidants, vitamins, and minerals. Seaweed snack packs may be used as a crunchy garnish for salads, soups, or rice bowls, or they can be enjoyed on their own as a fast and filling snack. Seaweed snacks have a distinct umami flavor that will definitely satisfy your cravings while being low in calories.

Creamy Cottage Cheese with Berries and Honey

For a sweet and creamy snack, top a serving of cottage cheese with a drizzle of honey and fresh fruit like raspberries, strawberries, or blueberries. Berries combine natural sweetness and antioxidants with cottage cheese's high protein and calcium content. Savor this simple and filling snack anytime of the day.

Popcorn

A light, crispy, high-fiber, low-calorie snack choice is air-popped popcorn. Savor unseasoned popcorn by itself or add flavor with a dash of nutritional yeast, sea salt, or your own spice combination. Popcorn is a satisfying snack that's ideal for movie nights, lunchtime cravings, or on-the-go nibbling.

Freeze-dried grapes

For hot summer days or whenever you're looking for something cool and refreshing, frozen grapes make a delightful and refreshing snack. Simply rinse and pat the grapes dry before freezing. Savor the naturally sweet and refreshing taste of frozen grapes straight from the freezer.

Rice Cake with Banana Slices and Almond Butter

For a filling and portable snack, spread almond butter over a rice cake and then place a sliced banana on top. The crispy basis is provided by rice cakes, while the protein and good fats come from almond butter. Slices of banana provide potassium and natural sweetness. This snack is ideal for giving you prolonged energy and satisfying your sweet needs

Bark with Greek Yogurt

After mixing Greek yogurt on a baking sheet covered with parchment paper after mixing it with a little amount of honey or maple syrup. Add your preferred nuts, seeds, granola, or fruits on top, and freeze until solid. After the yogurt bark has frozen, split it up into pieces and eat it as a wholesome and cool snack.

Slices of cucumber with tzatziki

Cut cucumber into rounds and serve with tzatziki sauce for a cool, zesty snack. Greek yogurt, cucumber, garlic, lemon juice, and herbs are combined to make the creamy and savory dip known as tzatziki sauce. Snacking on cucumber slices with tzatziki is a refreshing and light alternative.

Crackers made with whole grains and bean dip

To make a creamy bean dip, blend cooked beans (such as black beans, chickpeas, or white beans) with garlic, olive oil, lemon juice, and your preferred herbs and spices. Serve as a filling and high-protein snack with whole-grain crackers.

Bean dip is a satisfying and wholesome choice since it has fiber, protein, and complex carbs.

Nachos with apples

Cut apples into tiny circles and put them on a tray or plate. Spread peanut butter or almond butter over the surface, then top with dark chocolate chips, chopped nuts, dried fruit, and granola. Apple nachos are a unique and entertaining snack choice that's excellent for satisfying sweet tooths and packing in vital nutrients.

Chips with vegetables

Slice vegetables like sweet potatoes, beets, zucchini, or kale thinly and bake them in the oven until crispy to make your own veggie chips. For extra taste, season with sea salt, black pepper, or your preferred herbs and spices. Vegetable chips are a crispy and wholesome snack that's ideal for satisfying salty cravings.

Muffins with eggs

Beat eggs, cheese, veggies, and your preferred spices together to make a batch of egg muffins. Carefully spoon the mixture into the individual muffin cups and bake until it achieves a firm consistency. Egg muffins are a convenient, high-protein snack that's ideal for eating on the go. Warm or cold, egg muffins are a satisfying and substantial snack.

Ants in a Log

For a tasty and wholesome snack, spread almond or peanut butter on celery sticks and garnish with dried cranberries or raisins. Ants on a Log is a timeless childhood favorite that appeals to both children and adults. Savor this simple and filling snack anytime of the day.

Bell pepper slices with guacamole

Cut the bell peppers into strips and serve them with store-bought or homemade guacamole for a satisfyingly crunchy snack. Bell peppers are rich in antioxidants and vitamin C, while guacamole offers fiber and heart-healthy lipids. Savor this vibrant and nourishing snack whenever you're in the mood for something crunchy and savory.

Cups of Quinoa Salad

Once the quinoa is done, scoop it into little lettuce cups or hollow-out slices of cucumber, and top with your preferred salad toppings, including cherry tomatoes, cucumber, avocado, and feta cheese. Quinoa salad cups are a light and refreshing snack option that's perfect for an appetizer or afternoon pick-me-up.

Avocado with Chocolate Pudding

A smooth and creamy texture is achieved by blending ripe avocado with cocoa powder, honey or maple syrup, and a small amount of almond milk. Rich and decadent, chocolate avocado pudding is a snack choice that is full of antioxidants and beneficial fats. Savor this rich dessert or noon snack without feeling guilty. You can help your body burn fat, fill up on vital nutrients, and maintain consistent energy levels all day long by including these healthy snack ideas in your routine. To keep your snacks fresh and fulfilling, try experimenting with new taste combinations and ingredients.

Chapter 3

Formulating a Long-Term, Healthful Diet

● Planning and preparing meals

A healthy lifestyle and effective weight reduction depend heavily on meal planning and preparation. You can save time and money, cut down on food waste, and make sure you're choosing nutrient-dense foods that support your fitness and health objectives by taking the time to plan and prepare meals in advance. This section will discuss the advantages of meal planning and preparation, along with helpful hints and methods for getting started.

❖ **Advantages of Organizing and Preparing Meals**

- Encourages Healthy Eating: By organizing your meals, you may deliberately choose foods that are high in nutrients and provide well-balanced meals. You may promote general health and weight control by making sure your diet includes a mix of fruits, vegetables, whole grains, lean meats, and healthy fats. This can be achieved by organizing your meals in advance.

- Saves Time and Money: By lowering the need for impromptu grocery store runs or take away dinners, meal planning and preparation in advance may help you save both time and money. Making a grocery list and meal plan can expedite your shopping and prevent impulsive purchases. Furthermore, preparing meals at home is usually less expensive than going out to eat or getting takeout.

- Lessons Food Waste: By limiting your grocery shopping to the items you'll need for the next week, meal planning helps you avoid wasting or spoiling food. You can reduce food waste and maximize the use of your goods by organizing meals around components you already have on hand and coming up with inventive ways to repurpose leftovers.

- Supports Weight Reduction Objectives: By offering discipline and responsibility, meal planning and preparation in advance will help you maintain your weight reduction objectives. To avoid mindless eating and impulsive food choices, keep nutritious meals and snacks on hand. This will make it simpler to adhere to your calorie and nutritional targets.

- Encourages Variety and Creativity: Making a meal plan motivates you to experiment with different dishes, components, and taste combos, which results in a more intriguing and varied diet. By experimenting with various cuisines, cooking methods, and seasonal products, you may broaden your culinary knowledge and maintain an engaging and pleasurable mealtime experience.

❖ Useful Advice for Organizing and Preparing Meals

- Make Time for Planning: Set aside a certain amount of time every week to arrange your meals for the following week. This might take place on a Sunday afternoon or on any other day that best suits your plans. Take this time to plan your meals, look over recipes, and establish a shopping list.
- Start with the basics: Make basic, no-fuss meal plans that call for the fewest possible items and preparation time. To keep things interesting, try to balance the amounts of protein, carbs, and veggies in each meal. Aim for diversity.
- Make use of batch cooking: This method entails making a large amount of food at once and dividing it into portions for later meals. For simple meal assembly throughout the week, cook core components like grains, meats, and veggies in bulk and store them in separate containers in the fridge or freezer.
- Select versatile products: To increase productivity and cut down on waste, use products that can be utilized in a variety of dishes. For instance, roast a big batch of veggies and use them all week long in omelets, wraps, grain bowls, and salads.
- Prepare Ingredients Ahead of Time: To speed up the cooking process and save time throughout the week, wash, cut, and portion out ingredients beforehand. Meal assembly may be expedited and made easier by prepping components like fruits, vegetables, and grains in advance.

- Invest in Storage Containers: To preserve prepared items and leftovers, invest in a range of storage containers in various sizes and shapes. For simple reheating and cleaning, use glass or BPA-free plastic containers that are safe to use in the dishwasher and microwave.
- Label and Date Everything: To guarantee freshness and reduce food waste, label and date containers with the contents and the preparation date. To make it simple to identify products in the freezer or refrigerator, use detachable labels or masking tape.
- Make a Plan for Leftovers: Accept leftovers as a wholesome and practical choice for your next meal. Make extra food, and make a conscious effort to save leftovers for later in the week for lunch or supper. Use leftovers in creative ways, such as preparing new meals or adding them to grain bowls, salads, or wraps.
- Remain Flexible: Although meal planning may provide direction and structure, it's critical to maintain your flexibility and adaptability. As life changes and schedules change, be prepared to modify your meal plan as necessary and make replacements based on availability and preferences.
- Include the entire family: Ask your family for food suggestions, give them prep duties, and cook together to get everyone excited about the process of preparing meals. Meal planning with your family may promote healthy eating habits for all of you, while also fostering a sense of ownership and enthusiasm around mealtimes.

You must prepare balanced meals to maintain your general health, control your weight, and ensure that your body gets the nutrients it needs to flourish. A well-balanced meal has various macronutrients, such as proteins, fats, and carbs, and micronutrients, such as vitamins and minerals, to support body processes, provide energy, and enhance general health. The elements of a balanced meal, useful advice for creating balanced meals, and meal planning inspiration are all covered in this area.

→ Elements of a Well-Composed Meal

1. Protein: Protein is necessary for immunological response, muscular development and repair, hormone synthesis, and satiety. Meals that include a supply of lean protein boost metabolic health and muscular health while also helping you feel full and content. Lean meats (including chicken, turkey, fish, and lean cuts of cattle or pig), tofu, tempeh, legumes (such as beans, lentils, and chickpeas), eggs, dairy products, and plant-based protein powders are all excellent sources of protein.

2. Carbohydrates: The body uses carbohydrates as its main energy source and a source of vital nutrients, including fiber, vitamins, and minerals. Choose complex carbs from foods like whole grains (brown rice, quinoa, oats, barley, and whole wheat), starchy vegetables (sweet potatoes, potatoes, and winter squash), legumes, and fruits that are high in fiber and

low in added sugars. Including carbs in your meals promotes healthy blood sugar regulation, cognitive function, and bodily fuel.

3. Healthy Fats: Hormone balance, nutritional absorption, cognitive function, and satiety all depend on healthy fats. Including sources of heart-healthy fats in your meals may lower inflammation, boost overall wellbeing, and strengthen the heart. Pick unsaturated fats from foods like avocados, almonds, seeds, olive oil, coconut oil, and fatty fish like trout, salmon, and mackerel. Although fats are high in calories, watch how much you eat since they enhance taste, texture, and enjoyment.

4. Vegetables: Low in calories and rich in volume, vegetables are nutritional powerhouses that provide vital vitamins, minerals, antioxidants, and fiber. Non-starchy vegetables, including leafy greens, cruciferous vegetables (like broccoli, cauliflower, and Brussels sprouts), peppers, tomatoes, carrots, cucumbers, and zucchini, should make up half of your meal. You may be sure that you're receiving a wide range of nutrients and phytochemicals to promote general health by including a variety of colorful veggies in your meals.

5. Fruits: Adding sweetness and taste to meals and snacks, fruits are a natural source of vitamins, minerals, antioxidants, and fiber. Add whole fruits or fresh fruit slices as a nutrient-dense side dish or dessert to your meals. Try to get as much variety and taste as you can from your fruit intake; if at all feasible, use seasonal fruits to enhance their nutritional worth.

1. Apply the plate technique: To make sure your meals are wholesome and well-balanced, use the plate technique as a visual guide. Split your plate in half, then top one quarter with non-starchy veggies, another with healthy grains or lean protein, and the remaining quarter with non-starchy vegetables. Include a portion of fruit or dairy, as well as a serving of healthy fats, to complete your meal.

2. Plan Ahead: Give your weekly meal plans some thought, making sure to include a range of fruits, vegetables, grains, proteins, and fats in each dish. Make a shopping list of the products you'll need, and plan your meals using a meal planning template or app. Making a plan ahead of time guarantees that you have wholesome alternatives on hand and speeds up the cooking process.

3. Batch Cook: This method entails preparing a large amount of food at once and freezing it for later use. For simple weekly meal preparation, cook meats, grains, and veggies in large quantities and store them in separate containers in the fridge or freezer. In addition to saving time, batch cooking guarantees that you always have wholesome alternatives available.

4. Incorporate a Range of Colors and Textures: To make your meals visually attractive and fulfilling, try including a range of colors, textures, and tastes. To make your meals intriguing and delectable, try experimenting with various fruits, veggies,

grains, meats, herbs, and spices. You can be sure you're receiving a variety of nutrients and phytochemicals to promote optimum health when a vast assortment of foods is used.

5. Mind Your Portions: To avoid overindulging and to help achieve weight control objectives, be mindful of portion sizes. To portion out adequate serving quantities of protein, carbs, and fats, use measuring cups, food scales, or visual clues. To increase volume and fullness without adding extra calories, try to have half of your plate consist of non-starchy veggies.

6. Be flexible and adaptive: Although meal planning provides direction and structure, it's critical to remain adaptive and flexible. Be prepared to modify your meal plan as necessary and make replacements based on availability and preferences because life happens and schedules change. Accept leftovers as a healthy and practical alternative for your next meal.

7. Include Proteins from Plants: To add variety to your meals and cut down on saturated fats, try including plant-based protein sources like seitan, tofu, tempeh, edamame, and legumes (beans, lentils, and chickpeas). Rich in fiber, vitamins, minerals, and phytonutrients, plant-based proteins are a wholesome and sustainable choice for promoting general health.

8. Try Out Various Cooking Techniques: Use your imagination in the kitchen and try out various cooking techniques, including grilling, baking, roasting, steaming, sautéing, and stir-frying. Every cooking technique gives

components a distinct taste and texture, enabling you to make a range of mouthwatering and filling dishes. For a crunchy and savory twist, try air-frying or grilling veggies. For soft and succulent results, try slow-cooking meats and stews.

9. Add Flavor Without Adding Calories: Use herbs, spices, vinegar, citrus juice, and condiments like spicy sauce, mustard, and salsa to add flavor to your food without gaining additional calories. While spices like cumin, paprika, turmeric, and curry powder provide depth and complexity to meals, fresh herbs like basil, cilantro, parsley, and dill bring brightness and freshness. Try out a variety of flavor combinations to see which suits your palate the best.

10. Balance Your Plate Gradually: Although it's ideal to have balanced meals, it's OK if the plate approach isn't followed exactly every time. Rather, concentrate on maintaining a balance in your daily or weekly diet of macro- and micronutrients. To preserve balance and satiety, try to increase the amount of protein and healthy fats in your subsequent meal if your previous meal was higher in carbs.

→ **Instances of Well-Composed Meals**

1. Grilled Chicken Breast with Quinoa Salad and Steamed Broccoli: Quinoa salad contributes fiber and complex carbs; grilled chicken breast gives lean protein; and steaming broccoli adds vitamins, minerals, and antioxidants. For dessert, serve with a side of mixed berries.

2. Tofu, Brown Rice, and Mixed Vegetables in a Vegetarian Stir-Fry: Plant-based protein is provided by tofu, complex carbs are provided by brown rice, and fiber, vitamins, and minerals are added by mixed veggies. Tofu and veggies may be stir-fried in a tasty sauce and served over brown rice for a filling and healthy dinner.

3. Salmon Fillet with Sweet Potato Mash and Roasted Asparagus: Roasted asparagus contributes vitamins and minerals, sweet potato mash supplies fiber and complex carbs, and salmon offers protein and omega-3 fatty acids. Serve the salmon with a side of mixed green salad prepared with vinegar and olive oil, and sprinkle some lemon juice over it.

4. Turkey and Avocado Wrap with Whole Grain Tortilla and Mixed Green Salad: The whole grain tortilla provides fiber and complex carbs, while turkey supplies lean protein and healthy fats. Serve the wrap with a side of mixed green salad drizzled with balsamic vinaigrette and stuffed with sliced turkey, avocado, lettuce, tomato, and cucumber.

5. Vegetable Frittata with Whole Wheat Toast and Fresh Fruit Salad: A vegetable frittata gives fiber and complex carbs, while a fresh fruit salad contributes antioxidants, vitamins, and minerals. For a well-rounded and filling breakfast or brunch option, try the frittata with a side of mixed fruit salad and a piece of whole wheat bread.

6. Mediterranean Buddha Bowl:
The Mediterranean-inspired Buddha Bowl is a tasty and filling dish that combines a variety of tastes, textures, and

nutrients. Start with cooked quinoa or brown rice as the basis, then add grilled chicken or falafel on top for protein. Add a rainbow of vibrant veggies, including roasted eggplant, bell peppers, cucumbers, cherry tomatoes, and olives. Tahini dressing or tzatziki sauce may be drizzled over for more flavor and creaminess.

7. Bean and Vegetable Chili with Cornbread: During the colder months, bean and vegetable chili is a filling and satisfying dish. Put chopped tomatoes, onions, bell peppers, carrots, and celery in a saucepan with cooked beans (such as black beans, kidney beans, and pinto beans) and boil with chili spices until flavors blend. Savor a filling and healthy supper with a side of whole-grain cornbread for dunking.

8. Asian-Inspired Noodle Bowl: Packed with protein, veggies, and complex carbs, this Asian-inspired noodle bowl is a tasty and filling dinner alternative. Prepare soba noodles or rice noodles as directed on the box, and then mix in cooked shrimp, tofu, or tempeh along with a mix of veggies, including carrots, bell peppers, and mushrooms. Garnish with sesame seeds and green onions for extra flavor, then drizzle with a homemade or store-bought Asian-inspired sauce.

9. Quinoa Stuffed Bell Peppers: These colorful and nutrient-dense bell peppers are ideal for a quick lunch or supper. Prepare the quinoa per the directions on the box, then combine it with diced veggies, herbs, spices, and cooked ground turkey or black beans. Bake the filled bell peppers in halves until they are soft. For a full and well-balanced dinner, serve with steamed vegetables or a side salad.

10. Greek-Inspired Salad with Grilled Chicken: A Greek-inspired salad with grilled chicken is a light and refreshing dinner alternative, packed with flavor and taste. Begin with a bed of mixed greens, then top with feta cheese, cherry tomatoes, cucumber, red onion, and Kalamata olives. Add grilled chicken breast seasoned with oregano, garlic, and lemon juice over top, and for extra flavor, pour in Greek vinaigrette dressing.

- **Using Superfoods to Help Lose Weight**

Superfoods are nutrient-dense meals high in vitamins, minerals, antioxidants, and phytochemicals that help with weight reduction and provide a host of other health advantages. Superfoods help you regulate appetite, improve metabolism, get more critical nutrients, and feel better overall. To get these benefits, you can include them in your diet. This section will discuss the advantages of using superfoods in your diet to help you lose weight, as well as some popular superfoods to try and helpful meal and snack ideas.

→ Superfoods' Advantages for Losing Weight

1. Nutrient Density: Superfoods are comparatively low in calories but high in vital nutrients such as vitamins, minerals, antioxidants, and phytochemicals. By including superfoods in your diet, you can optimize your nutrient intake and minimize your calorie intake. This is crucial for promoting weight reduction and general wellness.

2. Increased levels of fiber, protein, and healthy fats found in many superfoods aid in promoting feelings of fullness and satiety, which in turn lessens the chance of overindulging and reaching for high-calorie, low-nutrient snacks. Superfoods may help you feel fuller for longer periods and have consistent energy levels throughout the day. Be sure to add these to your meals and snacks for a balanced diet.

3. Metabolism Boost: Certain superfoods feature ingredients that have been shown to raise fat burning and speed up metabolism, which may help with weight reduction attempts. For instance, the compound capsaicin found in chili peppers may boost calorie expenditure and decrease hunger, while catechins found in green tea have been shown to improve fat oxidation and speed up metabolism.

4. Blood Sugar Regulation: Research has shown that several superfoods, including berries, nuts, and leafy greens, may help control blood sugar levels and enhance insulin sensitivity. This is crucial for managing weight and lowering the risk of type 2 diabetes. By including these items in your diet, you can reduce cravings for sugary and high-carb meals and help stabilize blood sugar levels.

5. Anti-inflammatory effects: Because they are rich in antioxidants and phytochemicals, which lower inflammation in the body, many superfoods contain anti-inflammatory effects. Eating anti-inflammatory foods may help with weight reduction and general health since chronic inflammation has been connected to metabolic problems and obesity.

➔ **Well-liked Superfoods for Losing Weight**

1. Leafy Greens: Rich in vitamins, minerals, and antioxidants, leafy greens, such as kale, spinach, Swiss chard, and collard greens, are nutrient-dense superfoods with few calories. Including leafy greens in your meals and snacks helps you lose weight by providing satiety, water, and important nutrients.

2. Berries: Low in calories and sugar, berries, including strawberries, blueberries, raspberries, and blackberries, are a beneficial source of vitamins, fiber, and antioxidants. Berries are a wonderful option for low-calorie snacks, smoothies, and desserts since they bring sweetness and taste without increasing calorie intake.

3. Avocado: Packed with vitamins, minerals, fiber, and beneficial fats, avocados are a fruit that is high in nutrients. Avocados monounsaturated fats aid in satiety and feelings of fullness, while its fiber helps to maintain healthy digestion and blood sugar levels. Avocados are a delicious way to get important nutrients and add creaminess and richness to salads, sandwiches, and smoothies.

4. Salmon: Although it has comparatively few calories, salmon is a fatty fish that is high in protein, vitamins, and omega-3 fatty acids. It has been shown that omega-3 fatty acids aid in weight reduction by lowering inflammation, enhancing insulin sensitivity, and elevating sensations of

fullness. Eating salmon promotes satiety, general health, and the supply of vital nutrients.

5. Quinoa: Packed with protein, fiber, vitamins, and minerals, it is a gluten-free whole grain. Quinoa is a complete protein source because it has all nine necessary amino acids, unlike other grains. Quinoa's high protein and fiber composition assists in weight reduction objectives, provides sustained energy levels, and encourages feelings of fullness and satiety.

6. Greek Yogurt: Despite having comparatively few calories and sugar, Greek yogurt is a fantastic source of protein, calcium, and probiotics. Greek yogurt's protein aids in satiety and sensations of fullness, while its microorganisms aid in digestion and intestinal health. A wholesome and filling alternative for a snack or breakfast is plain Greek yogurt topped with your fruit, nuts, and seeds.

7. Chia Seeds: These little seeds are packed with fiber, protein, antioxidants, and omega-3 fatty acids. Chia seeds absorb liquids and turn into a gel-like substance when combined, which aids in promoting satiety and sensations of fullness. Chia seeds provide nourishment and help with weight reduction when added to salads, oats, smoothies, and yogurt.

8. Green Tea: Research has shown that the antioxidants in green tea, namely the catechins, might enhance metabolic processes and promote fat burning. Green tea is a widely consumed beverage. Regular use of green tea might enhance weight reduction efforts by augmenting caloric expenditure

and stimulating fat oxidation. Savor green tea as a calorie-free, revitalizing substitute for sweetened drinks.

9. Legumes: lentils are a fantastic source of fiber, vitamins, minerals, and plant-based protein. Legumes such as beans, lentils, and chickpeas are great examples of nutrient-rich foods to include in your diet. Legumes' high protein and fiber content supports blood sugar management, digestive health, and sensations of fullness and satisfaction. Legumes provide vital nutrients for your meals and snacks, as well as help you achieve your weight reduction goals.

10. Nuts and Seeds: Packed full of vitamins, minerals, protein, fiber, and healthy fats, nuts and seeds, including flaxseeds, walnuts, pumpkin seeds, and almonds, are foods high in nutrients. Nuts and seeds' healthy fats, protein, and fiber all work together to assist weight reduction objectives, provide sustained energy, and encourage feelings of fullness and satisfaction. Eat nuts and seeds as a snack or include them for an added nutritional boost in smoothies, cereal, yogurt, and salads.

→ **Useful Advice for Including Superfoods in Your Diet**

1. Start Slowly: As you become more familiar with superfoods, gradually increase your intake by starting with one or two at a time in your diet. Try out a variety of superfoods to see which ones suit your lifestyle and your taste buds.

2. Mix & Match: To optimize the nutritional value and taste of various superfoods, combine them in inventive and delectable ways. For instance, prepare a quinoa bowl with salmon, veggies, and chia seeds, or a kale salad with avocado, berries, and almonds. You can combine and mix superfoods to make a variety of wholesome and filling meals and snacks.

3. Snack Wisely: To increase your nutritional intake and support your weight reduction goals, swap out unhealthy snacks with ones based on superfoods. Snack on things like avocado toast with smoked salmon, Greek yogurt with berries and almonds, or a green smoothie with chia seeds, spinach, and banana. Superfood snacks provide you with the necessary nutrients to power your body in between meals and help you feel full.

4. Add to Daily Meals: To boost the nutritional content of your regular meals and dishes and aid in your weight reduction endeavors, use superfoods. To enhance taste and texture, you may, for instance, add spinach or kale to omelets, stir-fries, and pasta meals, or you can add berries and nuts to yogurt or oatmeal. Superfoods allow you to eat delicious and nutritious foods while also promoting your overall health and well-being.

5. Prepare ahead of time: Make superfood preparations and store them for easy access to fast meals and snacks. Berries, veggies, and leafy greens should all be cleaned, chopped, and kept in the refrigerator in sealed containers for quick access. Make a big pot of quinoa, beans, and lentils and dish them out for use all week long in salads, soups, and grain bowls. If they

are easier to add to your diet and stick to your weight reduction goals, they are ready to go.

6. Keep Yourself Hydrated: To keep hydrated and aid in your body's natural detoxification processes, sip plenty of water throughout the day. Water keeps you feeling full and content in between meals and aids in the removal of waste and toxins from the body. Try to have eight glasses of water or more each day, and for extra taste and freshness, add slices of cucumber or lemon.

7. Listen to Your Body: Be aware of how different superfoods make your body feel, and constantly adjust your intake. Since each person has different dietary requirements and preferences, it's important to pay attention to your body's signals of hunger and fullness and eat consciously. If some superfoods make you queasy, try others or limit your intake.

8. Change items: To improve the nutritional value and help you reach your weight reduction objectives, swap out less nutritious items in your favorite dishes with superfoods. For instance, in baking recipes, swap out white rice for cauliflower rice, pasta for zucchini noodles, and flour for almond or coconut flour. By substituting components, you can still enjoy your favorite recipes while making them healthier and more conducive to weight reduction.

9. Blend superfoods into smoothies for a handy and quick approach to boost your vitamin intake and help you reach your weight reduction objectives. For a nutrient-dense and filling lunch or snack, try adding protein powder, berries,

avocado, chia seeds, and leafy greens like spinach or kale to your favorite smoothie recipes. Smoothies are a wonderful way to include superfoods in your diet since they are adaptable and flexible.

10. Use Superfoods as Toppings: To add taste, texture, and nutritional value to yogurt, oats, salads, soups, and other meals, sprinkle superfoods on top. For a little crunch and sweetness, top yogurt with berries, nuts, and seeds. For an additional nutritious boost, sprinkle chia, hemp, or flax seeds over salads, soups, or stir-fries. With superfoods as toppings, you can improve the flavor and nutritional content of your meals without consuming more calories.

11. Try New Superfood Recipes: To broaden your culinary horizons and assist with weight reduction objectives, experiment with new recipes and cooking methods that highlight superfoods as the main component. Search for dishes that creatively and delectably use superfoods like quinoa, chia seeds, kale, and salmon on the internet, in cookbooks, or on food blogs. Try varying the flavor combinations and cooking techniques to find new, delicious, and healthy favorite recipes.

12. Combine Superfoods with Protein: To produce balanced, filling meals that promote muscle development and repair while encouraging weight reduction, pair superfoods with lean protein sources like chicken, turkey, fish, tofu, or beans. For a wholesome and filling supper, try adding baked fish and roasted veggies to quinoa or combining grilled chicken and avocado with kale salad. Protein and superfoods work

together to assist your weight reduction goals by keeping you feeling full and content.

→ **Superfood-Boosted Meal Examples.**

1. Berry Spinach Smoothie: For a nutrient-dense and filling breakfast or snack alternative, blend spinach, mixed berries, banana, Greek yogurt, and chia seeds with almond milk. This smoothie will help you reach your weight reduction objectives and maintain an energy level throughout the day since it is full of vitamins, minerals, antioxidants, protein, and fiber.

2. Salmon Quinoa Salad: For a vibrant and wholesome salad that's ideal for lunch or supper, combine cooked quinoa with flaked salmon, mixed greens, avocado, cherry tomatoes, cucumber, and pumpkin seeds. This salad is a filling and weight-loss-friendly lunch choice since it's high in protein, fiber, healthy fats, vitamins, and minerals.

3. Kale and Berry Salad: To make a delectable and nutrient-rich salad that is bursting with color and taste, combine chopped kale, mixed berries, walnuts, goat cheese, and balsamic vinaigrette. In addition to pleasing your palate, this salad's abundance of vitamins, antioxidants, fiber, and healthy fats can help you reach your weight reduction objectives.

4. Quinoa-Stuffed Bell Peppers: For a tasty and wholesome suppertime dish, stuff half bell peppers with cooked quinoa, black beans, corn, diced tomatoes, avocado, and cilantro.

These filling and weight-loss-friendly stuffed peppers are high in fiber, protein, vitamins, and minerals.

5. Chia Seed Pudding: To thicken into a creamy pudding-like consistency, combine chia seeds, almond milk, vanilla essence, and a little amount of honey or maple syrup. Refrigerate the mixture overnight. For a healthy and filling dessert or snack, sprinkle some honey, sliced almonds, and fresh berries on top. Rich in fiber, protein, antioxidants, and omega-3 fatty acids, chia seed pudding is a nutritious and weight-loss-friendly dessert.

- **Tips for Eating Out**

While eating out may be simple and pleasurable, it can also be difficult to stick to a nutritious diet and support weight reduction objectives. You can, however, browse restaurant menus and choose healthier options while still enjoying delectable meals if you use certain thoughtful decision-making techniques. This section will provide helpful advice for eating out, such as mindful eating techniques, portion management techniques, and healthier menu choices.

➤ **Choosing Healthier Menu Items**

1. Examine the Menu Ahead of Time: If at all feasible, spend some time looking over the menu online before visiting the restaurant. Seek out selections that are richer in veggies, whole grains, lean protein, and less in calories, saturated fat, and salt. Nowadays, a lot of eateries provide healthier menu

choices or use labels or symbols to show which selections are lighter.

2. Choose grilled, steaming, or baking options Choose dishes that are baked, steamed, or grilled from the menu instead of fried or breaded. These cooking techniques are often healthier options since they have less added fat and calories. Instead of fried or creamy side dishes, go for baked potatoes, steamed rice, fish, and grilled chicken.

3. Ask for Changes: Don't be scared to request that menu items be changed to a healthier version. Ask to have meals made with less oil or butter, request side orders of sauces, dressings, and toppings so you can manage how much you use, or ask to have higher-calorie items replaced with healthier options (e.g., whole grain bread instead of white bread, brown rice instead of white rice).

4. Emphasize Lean Proteins and Vegetables: Center your dinner around a variety of lean protein sources, like grilled chicken, fish, tofu, or lentils, as well as a large serving of vegetables. Foods high in protein and fiber are essential for promoting feelings of fullness and satisfaction during meals, which makes them ideal for weight reduction. Choose salads, soups made with vegetables, or side dishes as your main course or as a way to get more veggies in your diet.

5. Be Aware of Portions: When placing an order, be mindful of the portion sizes and think about splitting an entrée or, if smaller portions are available, choosing them. Since restaurant servings are usually greater than those of a regular

home meal, try to eat until you're full rather than clearing your plate. Consider using an appetizer or side salad as your main dish, or box up half of your meal to go.

> ➤ **Applying Portion Management**

1. Use Your Hand as a Guide: When eating out, use your hand as a general reference for portion sizes. The size of your palm should represent the approximate amount of protein you eat; your fist should represent the approximate amount of carbs, such as rice or pasta; and your clenched fist should represent the approximate amount of vegetables you eat. You don't have to measure or weigh your food to determine the right portion amounts using this easy approach.

2. Start with a Salad or Vegetable Soup: To help you feel fuller with meals high in nutrients while controlling your calorie consumption, start your meal with a salad or vegetable-based soup. Selecting a salad or soup with plenty of vegetables and a broth base can help you control your hunger and avoid overindulging in the main dish.

3. Share meals or order appetizers: To reduce portion sizes and calories, think about splitting meals with your dining partners or ordering appetizers in place of your main dish. Smaller portion sizes or appetizer alternatives are available at many restaurants, and they may be just as filling as a full dinner. You can sample a variety of menu items while also controlling portion sizes by sharing dishes.

4. Request a To-Go Box: When your food is provided, don't be afraid to request a to-go box if it arrives in large servings. As soon as possible, portion out a smaller serving size for yourself and save the remainder for a later meal. Adopting this approach can help you steer clear of mindless eating while allowing you to relish your preferred restaurant dishes without going overboard.

1.3 Using Mindful Food Practices

1. Eat slowly and mindfully: Give your food your full attention while taking your time to appreciate all of its tastes, textures, and scents. Eating slowly reduces the risk of overeating by allowing your body to register feelings of contentment and fullness. In between mouthfuls, put down your fork, converse with your dining partners, and observe your body's signals of hunger and fullness.

2. Pay Attention to Your Body: Recognize when your body is hungry and full, and eat until you're content but not too full. You should stop eating, even if there is food left on your plate when you are pleasantly satisfied. Remind yourself that it's OK to take leftovers home for another meal or to leave food behind.

3. Remain Hydrated: To keep hydrated and feel fuller throughout your meal, sip water. Drinking water in between bites might help avoid overindulging in food since sometimes thirst can be confused with hunger. Drinks low in calories, such as water, sparkling water, or unsweetened tea, are preferable to drinks high in sugar or alcohol.

4. Practice Portion Distortion Awareness: Pay attention to dish sizes and steer clear of the often-observed excessive portions at restaurants. If your portion is too big, don't feel obligated to eat it all. Use visual cues to help you determine the right portion sizes and avoid overindulging, such as comparing the size of your meal to the size of your hand.

5. Savor the Experience: Going out to eat is about more than simply the cuisine. While eating, pay attention to the company you have, the restaurant's atmosphere, and the opportunity to sample new dishes and sensations. Remind yourself that one decadent meal won't ruin your attempts to lose weight, so feel free to savor the occasion.

Chapter 4

Losing Weight and Hydration

- **Water's Critical Role in Weight Management**

Although water is sometimes disregarded as a crucial element of an effective weight-management plan, its benefits for both weight reduction and general health cannot be overemphasized. Numerous physiological functions in the body, such as metabolism, digestion, hunger control, and energy generation, depend on maintaining an appropriate level of hydration. This section will discuss the importance of water in weight management, the benefits of maintaining hydration, achievable strategies for increasing water consumption, and the possible negative effects of dehydration on weight loss attempts.

★ **Metabolism and hydration**

1. Water is essential for metabolism, which is the process by which your body turns food into energy. Water is a component of every metabolic process in the body, so maintaining enough hydration is critical for proper metabolic function. Maintaining a healthy weight depends on effective energy

generation, nutrition absorption, and waste disposal, all of which are supported by drinking enough water.

2. Water consumption has been shown to enhance the body's calorie burning, or energy expenditure. The body attempts to bring water to body temperature after ingestion, a process known as "water-induced thermogenesis," which causes a brief rise in calorie burning. Even though attempts may not have had an impact, metabolism is excellent; every little bit helps with weight control initiatives.

★ Controlling Appetite and Feeling Full

1. Before meals, water has been shown to help suppress appetite and lower calorie consumption. According to studies, drinking water before meals may boost feelings of fullness and decrease sensations of hunger, which can reduce the number of calories consumed during the meal. For anyone trying to cut down on calories overall and manage portion sizes, this simple method might be quite beneficial.

2. Satiety: Maintaining hydration levels in between meals may also aid in fostering a sense of fullness or satiety. Sometimes people confuse dehydration for hunger, which results in overindulging in unneeded snacks. You can eventually achieve weight-control goals by drinking enough water throughout the day to prevent mindless snacking and cravings.

★ Metabolism and Absorption of Nutrients

1. Digestive Health: Water plays an important role in proper digestion and nutrition absorption. Drinking enough water enables the digestive system to soften and break down food, allowing the body to absorb nutrients and expel waste more easily. Drinking enough water can help avoid constipation, bloating, and other digestive problems that may impede attempts to control weight.

2. Nutrient Transport: The movement of nutrients throughout the body is facilitated by water. After being absorbed by the digestive system, nutrients are transported to cells and tissues via circulation. Maintaining enough hydration ensures effective nutrient transport, allowing vital nutrients to arrive at their correct locations and facilitating a variety of metabolic functions.

★ Vitality and Structural Efficiency

1. Energy Production: The body needs water to produce energy. Dehydration can lead to feelings of weariness, sluggishness, and impaired physical and mental functioning. By ensuring that your body gets the fluids it needs to create energy effectively, being properly hydrated helps you feel focused, awake, and invigorated all day long.

2. Exercise Performance: Drinking enough water is essential for both optimum exercise output and quick recovery. Dehydration raises the risk of heat-related disorders, including heat exhaustion and heat strokes, and may decrease endurance, strength, and coordination, all of which can negatively impact physical performance. Water consumption

before, during, and after exercise supports electrolyte balance, prevents dehydration, and promotes peak performance and recuperation.

★ Useful Advice for Increasing Water Consumption

1. Establish a water intake goal. Make sure you're keeping well hydrated; try to drink a certain quantity of water every day. Although the amount of water required for each person varies depending on age, weight, activity level, and climate, it is generally advised to consume at least 16 glasses of water, or around 4 liters, every day. Adapt your diet to your individual needs and lifestyle.

2. Maintain Water Accessibility: Carry a reusable water bottle with you wherever you go to make it simple to grab water throughout the day. Having water on hand makes it easier to remember to remain hydrated, whether you're at home, at work, at school, or on the move. Pick a water bottle that you want to use that is simple to carry around, and fill it up as required throughout the day.

3. Water Before Meals: To help suppress hunger and avoid overindulging, make it a practice to have a glass of water before every meal. Not only can drinking water before meals make you feel fuller, but it also guarantees that you are well hydrated before starting your meal. Have a glass of water 30 minutes before eating to maximize its hunger-reduction effects.

4. Natural Water Flavoring: If you're not a fan of plain water, try adding some fresh fruit, herbs, or vegetables to naturally flavor it. For a tasty and refreshing touch to your water that doesn't include any extra sugar or calories, add slices of lemon, lime, cucumber, or berries. Try a variety of taste combinations until you discover ones that you like and eagerly anticipate sipping all day.

5. Eat Hydrating Foods: In addition to drinking water, you can increase your fluid intake by eating high-water-content items such as fruits and vegetables. Numerous fruits and vegetables are rich in water and may help you stay hydrated overall. Oranges, lettuce, cucumbers, strawberries, watermelon, and strawberries are hydrating foods that may increase your fluid consumption.

6. Set Reminders: To help you remember to drink water throughout the day, set alarms or reminders on your computer or phone. You can plan specific times throughout the day to drink a glass of water or set a timer to go off every hour to remind you to take a sip. You may be more certain that you're hitting your water consumption targets if you prioritize staying hydrated and include it in your daily routine.

7. Monitor Your Intake: Use a notebook, an app, or a wearable gadget to keep track of how much water you drink each day. You can identify patterns or trends in your hydration habits and maintain accountability by keeping an eye on how much water you drink. Instead of attempting to consume a lot of water at once, consider spreading it out evenly throughout the day.

★ Possible Effects of Dehydration on Attempts to Lose Weight

1. Dehydration may impede metabolic processes and reduce the body's ability to burn calories, resulting in decreased energy expenditure and difficulty losing weight. Dehydration may cause the body to slow down metabolic processes in an attempt to preserve energy, which might impede weight reduction attempts by lowering energy expenditure.

2. Increased Appetite and Cravings: Dehydration may sometimes be misinterpreted for hunger, which results in an increase in appetite and a desire for meals rich in calories and energy. This may lead to overindulging and ingesting too many calories, which might undermine attempts to lose weight. By avoiding hunger and desires brought on by dehydration, being well hydrated helps you choose better foods.

3. Reduced Endurance, Strength, and Coordination: Dehydration may lead to a reduction in endurance, strength, and coordination during physical activity. It can also raise the risk of tiredness and injury. Exercise becomes more difficult and less beneficial for promoting weight reduction when the body is dehydrated. To maximize calorie burning and performance, it's critical to be well hydrated before, during, and after exercise.

4. Water Retention: In a paradoxical way, the body's effort to preserve fluids in reaction to dehydration may sometimes

result in water retention. This may lead to bloating and a transient weight increase, which might conceal real fat reduction and demotivate people to keep trying to lose weight. Drinking enough water has two benefits: maintaining proper fluid balance in the body and preventing water retention due to dehydration.

5. Impaired Fat Metabolism: Losing too much water may make it more difficult for the body to properly metabolize fat for energy, which can make it more difficult to lose weight. Because water is involved in the breakdown and transport of fatty acids for energy generation, proper fat metabolism requires enough hydration. Because fat metabolism may be affected, the body may use less of its stored fat as a fuel source when it is dehydrated.

6. Changed Hormone Levels: The body's hormone levels, especially those governing hunger, metabolism, and fluid balance, may be upset by dehydration. Dehydration may cause increases in the hunger hormone ghrelin and reductions in the satiety hormone leptin, according to research. This can lead to increased sensations of hunger and decreased feelings of fullness. Moreover, dehydration may change insulin, cortisol, and other hormone levels that are involved in metabolism and weight control, making weight reduction attempts even more difficult.

7. Water weight reduction vs. fat loss: When tracking your weight loss progress, it's critical to make a distinction between the two types of weight loss. Changes in fluid balance brought on by dehydration or fluctuations in hydration status may

result in brief variations in body weight; however, these changes may not be indicative of actual fat loss. Even though rapid weight loss from water may initially appear on the scale, it is neither sustainable nor a sign of long-term fat reduction. To encourage healthy, long-lasting fat reduction, focus your attention on making small, sustainable changes to your diet and lifestyle.

★ Recommendations for Hydration in Weight Management

1. Track Urine Color: Keeping an eye on the color of your urine is a quick and easy method to determine your level of hydration. While deeper yellow or amber-colored urine may suggest dehydration, pale yellow or straw-colored pee often indicates appropriate hydration. To maintain a light yellow tint, make sure you drink water often throughout the day.

2. Weigh yourself often: To monitor changes in body weight over time, weigh yourself frequently under regular circumstances, such as first thing in the morning before eating or drinking. Remember that changes in weight are common and may be caused by a variety of variables, including food consumption, activity, and level of hydration. Pay more attention to long-term patterns than to daily variations.

3. Listen to Your Body: Whenever you feel thirsty, note your body's cues and sip water. In order to avoid dehydration, it is important to swiftly address thirst as a trustworthy signal of hydration status. Furthermore, emphasize drinking water

when you see symptoms of dehydration, such as headaches, lethargy, dark urine, dry mouth, and dizziness.

4. Drink Throughout the Day: To maintain optimum levels of hydration, try to drink water regularly throughout the day instead of attempting to "catch up" on it all at once. Drinking water frequently replaces fluids lost through perspiration, breathing, and sweating, particularly after meals and physical exercise.

5. Consider fluids: Adjust your fluid intake according to your age, weight, exercise level, climate, and personal hydration requirements. You can increase your fluid intake by including non-alcoholic beverages like herbal tea, sparkling water, and high-hydration meals in addition to water. Pay attention to fluid loss when it's hot outside, when you're exercising hard, or in other circumstances when you require more fluids.

6. Recognize Hydration Challenges: There are a few things that may make it harder to keep well hydrated and raise the risk of dehydration. These include excessive heat, altitude, strenuous activity, sickness, using prescription drugs, and drinking alcohol. In these circumstances, take proactive steps to stay hydrated by increasing your fluid intake and keeping a close eye on your hydration level.In summaryWater is essential for maintaining a healthy weight and general well-being. Maintaining a healthy weight requires regulating metabolism, hunger, digestion, nutritional absorption, energy levels, and exercise performance—all of which are aided by drinking enough water. You can support your weight management efforts and advance your overall health and

well-being by making hydration a priority and implementing helpful strategies for boosting water consumption into your daily routine.

- **Drinks That Rehydrate and Their Substitutes**

Although water is the ideal beverage for hydration, there are many additional options that might increase your fluid consumption. Maintaining proper hydration is crucial for general health and wellbeing. This section will discuss some hydrating drinks and substitutes, their possible advantages and disadvantages, and how to include them in a well-balanced hydration regimen.

→ **Water is the best source of hydration.**

The most basic and important beverage for staying hydrated is water. It has no calories, is widely accessible, and is essential for many bodily physiological processes. Throughout the day, it's essential to consume enough water to stay hydrated, promote metabolism, aid with digestion, and control body temperature.

Advantages of Water

- Delivers vital hydration without the addition of calories, sweets, or artificial substances.
- Promotes the best possible metabolism and energy generation.
- Promotes nutrition absorption and digestion.

- Aids in controlling body temperature and guards against overheating while exercising.
- Encourages satiety and fullness sensations, which may support attempts to control weight.

Taking into account

- Each person has different demands for water depending on their age, weight, activity level, climate, and general health.Try to stay hydrated by drinking water often throughout the day, as opposed to waiting until you're feeling parched.
- Keep an eye out for thirst signals and urine color, which are indicators of your level of hydration. Adjust your fluid intake accordingly.

➔ **Herbal Tea: rich in flavor and low in calories**

Since they don't include extra calories or caffeine and come in a range of flavors, herbal teas are a well-liked substitute for regular water. Depending on personal inclination, herbal teas may be sipped hot or cold and are prepared with dried herbs, flowers, fruits, or spices.

The advantages of herbal tea

- Offers taste and diversity in addition to hydration.
- Offer potential health benefits based on the herbs and other ingredients used.

- It's naturally caffeine-free, so it's beneficial for anyone who is sensitive to the stimulant or wants to cut down on their consumption.
- It is a versatile option that suits a variety of tastes and preferences because it can be consumed hot or cold.

Taking into account

- Carefully read ingredient labels to steer clear of teas that have artificial flavors, extra sugars, or other ingredients.
- Try out several herbal tea blends to discover tastes and combinations that you like.
- To maintain quality and ingredient control, try making herbal tea at home using loose leaf tea or tea bags.

→ Coconut Water: A Natural Electrolyte Source

As a natural electrolyte supply and hydrating beverage, coconut water has grown in popularity, especially among athletes and physically active people. Young green coconuts contain a transparent liquid called "coconut water," which is naturally high in electrolytes including potassium, sodium, and magnesium.

Coconut water advantages

- It provides hydration by replenishing electrolytes lost through perspiration during exercise or in hot conditions.

- Naturally contains calcium, sodium, and magnesium. These electrolytes are necessary for maintaining fluid balance, hydration, and muscular performance.
- It's a calorie-efficient, naturally sweet substitute for sugary sports drinks that's also hydrating.
- Has trace levels of antioxidants, vitamins, and minerals that may provide further health advantages.

Taking into account

- Coconut water should be used in moderation, particularly if one is managing their calorie or sugar consumption, since it may contain more natural sugars than regular water.
- For the healthiest alternative, look for coconut water products that don't include any artificial additives or extra sugars.
- Although coconut water has some health benefits, it shouldn't usually take the place of regular water as the main source of hydration.

→ **Infused Water: Tasty and adaptable**

To add taste and nutrition to simple water, fruits, vegetables, herbs, or spices are added. This process is called infused water, often referred to as fruit-infused water or spa water. A nourishing and refreshing beverage alternative, infused water may be tailored with a broad range of substances to fit personal preferences and tastes.

The benefits of infused water

- Enhances the taste and attractiveness of plain water by adding natural flavor and diversity.
- Offers a mild source of antioxidants, vitamins, and minerals from fruits, vegetables, and herbs.has no artificial additives or added sugars, making it a calorie-free, healthy substitute for sweetened drinks.
- Can be quickly and simply made at home using frozen or fresh produce, fruits, and herbs, opening up many taste options and creative possibilities.

Taking into account

- Try a variety of fruit, vegetable, and herb combinations until you discover a taste you like.For optimal flavor infusion, let the infused water soak in the refrigerator for a few hours or overnight.
- Use a reusable infuser container or pitcher to retain the solid components, or strain them out before drinking.

→ **Drinks that replenish electrolytes:**

Electrolyte drinks are designed to replace the fluids and electrolytes lost during strenuous exercise, perspiration, or physical activity. They are often referred to as sports drinks or rehydration drinks. Water, electrolytes (such as sodium, potassium, and magnesium), carbohydrates, and sometimes flavorings or sweeteners are the usual ingredients of these drinks.

Electrolyte beverage benefits:

- Resupplies fluids and electrolytes lost via perspiration during vigorous physical activity, hot weather, and exercise.
- Supports the maintenance of muscle tone, fluid balance, and hydration during extended or intense activity sessions.
- Offers a readily absorbed supply of carbohydrates for energy during longer-than-60-minute endurance exercises.
- May include electrolytes in ratios and concentrations that are best for hydration and functionality.

Taking into account

- Electrolyte drinks may not be required for regular hydration requirements; instead, they are often meant to be consumed during extended or strenuous activity.
- For the healthiest choice, choose electrolyte drinks without artificial chemicals or additional sweets.If you use electrolyte drinks for hydration outside of high-intensity workout scenarios, consider diluting them with water to reduce the amount of sugar and calories.

→ Sparkling Water: Delightful and revitalizing

A solution of water that has been pressure-infused with carbon dioxide gas to produce bubbles and effervescence is called sparkling water, often referred to as carbonated water or soda water. Sparkling water, which has a frothy texture and a variety of tastes without extra calories or sugar, is a well-liked and cooling substitute for regular water.

The benefits of sparkling water

Offers hydration, extra fizz, and texture for a delightful and rejuvenating beverage experience.
Available in a variety of flavors to accommodate a range of tastes and preferences, including unsweetened and natural fruit flavors.
Because it is low-calorie and sugar-free, it is a healthier alternative to sugar-filled sodas, soft drinks, and other carbonated beverages since it is low in calories and sugar-free.
Tastes good on its own or as a foundation for mocktails, mixed cocktails, and flavored beverages.

Taking into account

For the healthiest option, choose naturally flavored or unsweetened sparkling water that doesn't include artificial sweeteners or additional sugars.
Watch out for flavored sparkling drinks that may contain artificial sweeteners, added sugars, or other ingredients that increase calorie and sugar consumption.
Use still water or other non-carbonated drinks if you are sensitive to carbonation or are feeling queasy in your stomach.

In conclusion, a variety of hydrating drinks and substitutes are available to help you meet your fluid requirements and hydration objectives. Even though water is the best way to stay hydrated, you may spice up your hydration regimen with different alternatives, including herbal tea, coconut water, infused water, electrolyte drinks, and sparkling water. There are several alternatives available, whether your goal is to keep hydrated all day, enjoy a flavor-infused beverage after working out, or restore electrolytes after an intense workout. You can maintain proper hydration and promote your general health and well-being by including a variety of hydrating drinks in your daily routine and being aware of added sugars and artificial substances.

- **Tips for Hydration in Weight Loss**

Not only is drinking enough water important for overall health, but it also helps promote weight reduction goals.

Achieving and maintaining a healthy weight depends on a number of aspects, including improved digestion, increased metabolism, hunger regulation, and improved exercise performance when drinking enough water. We'll look at several hydration strategies in this part that are especially designed to help you stay hydrated while losing weight.

1. Make water consumption a priority.

Water is the most hydrating beverage available and ought to be your go-to option for keeping hydrated, particularly if you're attempting to reduce weight. Water contains no calories, sugar, or chemicals that may impede weight loss, unlike sugar-filled drinks and artificially flavored beverages.

Making water intake a priority allows you to stay well hydrated throughout the day without gaining too much weight or sacrificing your health goals.

2. Establish hydration objectives.

Establishing hydration targets can assist you in sticking to your weight reduction plan. As a general rule, try to consume eight 8-ounce glasses (or around 2 liters) of water per day. Individual water requirements, however, could differ depending on things like environment, activity level, weight, and age. To keep track of your daily water consumption and make sure you're constantly reaching your hydration goals, think about utilizing a notebook or water monitoring app.

3. Prior to meals, sip water.

Water consumption before meals is a useful weight-loss tactic because it helps reduce hunger and prevent overeating. Thirty minutes before meals, drinking a glass of water will help you feel fuller and consume fewer calories throughout the meal. Furthermore, drinking enough water before meals might prevent thirst from being confused with hunger and result in overindulging in snacks or meals. To help you lose weight, make it a habit to have a glass of water before every meal.

4. Keep a reusable water bottle with you.

One useful technique to ensure you have access to water throughout the day is to always carry a reusable water bottle with you. Water assists you to stay hydrated and avoids dehydration, whether you're exercising, doing errands, or at work. To maintain adequate hydration levels throughout the day, choose a BPA-free water bottle that you enjoy using and find convenient to carry, and refill it as needed.

5. Naturally Tasty Water

If you don't like the taste of plain water, try adding some natural flavoring, such as fresh fruits, vegetables, or herbs. You may add flavor and enjoyment to your water by adding slices of lemon, lime, cucumber, berries, or mint. Try a variety of taste combinations until you discover ones that you like and eagerly anticipate sipping all day. To keep flavored water calorie-free and nutritious, don't add sugar syrups, artificial sweeteners, or other additions.

6. Consume foods that are hydrating.

To enhance your fluid intake and maintain hydration, include hydrating items in your diet in addition to drinking water. Due to their high water content, many fruits and vegetables may help you meet your recommended daily consumption of fluids. Examples of hydrating foods are watermelon, cucumbers, strawberries, oranges, lettuce, and celery. These foods also include vital minerals and fiber to help you stay hydrated. To maintain your hydration and satisfaction levels throughout the day, include a variety of hydrating foods in your meals and snacks.

7. Check the color of your urine.

Keeping an eye on the color of your pee might provide important information about your level of hydration. A straw-colored or light yellow urine indicates that you are well hydrated. Urine that is more amber or darker in color might indicate dehydration, which means you need to consume more water. To maintain ideal levels of hydration, monitor the color of your urine throughout the day and modify the amount of fluid you consume accordingly. Urine color may be affected by some drugs, meals, and supplements, so use it as a general guideline rather than a reliable measure of your level of hydration.

8. Do not consume caloric beverages.

Drinks high in calories, such as alcoholic beverages, sugary drinks, and caffeinated coffee or tea, should be avoided because they may cause weight gain and undermine your attempts to lose weight. As your main source of hydration, choose water or sugar-free drinks to cut down on extra calories and additional sugars. If you want flavored beverages, go for the unsweetened varieties or naturally flavor water with spices, herbs, or fruits to make it low in calories and nutritious.

9. Drink plenty of water while exercising.

Sufficient hydration is crucial for maintaining fluid equilibrium, controlling body temperature, and promoting peak performance while exercising. Before, during, and after exercise, sip water to replace fluids lost via perspiration and avoid becoming dehydrated. Depending on individual sweat rates and activity intensity, the American College of Sports Medicine suggests consuming 16–20 ounces of water two to three hours before exercise, 8–10 ounces 10–20 minutes before exercise, and 7–10 ounces every 10–20 minutes during exercise.

10. Pay attention to your body.

Most importantly, pay attention to your body's thirst signals and sip water whenever you sense them. In order to avoid dehydration, it is important to swiftly address thirst as a trustworthy signal of hydration status. Additionally, emphasize drinking water when you see symptoms of dehydration, such as headaches, lethargy, dark urine, dry mouth, and dizziness. To assist your weight reduction efforts, pay attention to your body's cues and prioritize staying hydrated throughout the day.

11. Create a hydration plan in advance.

If you plan ahead and prioritize being hydrated, you may include it in your everyday routine. Always have a water bottle with you; set alerts to remind you to stay hydrated throughout the day; and include hydration planning in your meal and snack schedule. By making being hydrated a mindful habit, you can guarantee that you're always meeting your fluid requirements and advancing your weight reduction goals.

12. Maintain consistency

When it comes to weight reduction and hydration, consistency is essential. By including drinking water in your daily routine and adhering to your hydration objectives, you may develop the habit of drinking it. Make being hydrated a top priority and an essential component of your daily routine, whether you're at home, at work, or on the road. You may enhance your weight reduction efforts, boost your metabolism, and maintain appropriate fluid balance by adhering to a rigorous hydration regimen.

Sufficient hydration is crucial for effective weight reduction. You can maximize hydration and support your weight loss goals by making water consumption a priority, setting hydration goals, drinking water before meals, carrying a reusable water bottle, naturally flavoring hydrating, eating hydrating foods, keeping an eye on the color of your urine, avoiding liquid calories, staying hydrated during exercise, paying attention to your body's thirst cues, planning ahead for hydration, and being consistent with your hydration habits. To keep hydrated, motivated, and on track with your weight reduction quest, include these useful hydration techniques into your daily routine.

Chapter 5

Managing Stress to Lose

Although stress is a normal reaction to difficult circumstances, chronic or sustained stress may have serious negative effects on one's general health, including the ability to control one's weight. Stress is an inherent part of life. This section delves into the intricate correlation between stress and weight gain, including the physiological processes implicated, the psychological aspects under consideration, and pragmatic approaches to stress management that bolster weight reduction objectives.

1. The Body's Reaction to Stress

Your body releases chemicals like cortisol and adrenaline as part of the "fight or flight" reaction when it experiences stress, regardless of the source—work, relationships, money, or anything else. These stress hormones raise blood pressure, heart rate, and energy availability to prime the body to react to perceived threats. While in acute or short-term conditions this reaction is necessary for survival, persistent stress may cause the stress response system to become dysregulated, which can have negative implications on metabolism, hunger control, and weight management.

2. Cortisol and Gaining Weight

Known as the "stress hormone," cortisol regulates metabolism, energy balance, and fat storage in addition to being a key player in the body's reaction to stress. Chronic stress may cause cortisol levels to stay high for extended periods, which can cause appetite dysregulation, cravings for high-calorie meals, increased fat deposition, and abdominal obesity. Studies have shown that those who experience or perceive higher levels of chronic stress are more likely to have elevated cortisol levels, which increases the likelihood of weight gain or difficulty losing weight.

3. Dysregulation of Appetite

Prolonged stress may cause abnormalities in hunger, satiety, and food choices, which can lead to weight gain by upsetting the body's mechanism that controls appetite. Some people may have a reduced appetite or have lost interest in eating as a coping technique for stress, while others may have increased hunger and a desire for high-calorie, high-sugar items. Developing healthier eating habits can help prevent overeating, emotional eating, and irregular eating patterns, ultimately supporting weight management..

4. Emotional eating and food cravings

Emotional eating habits are brought on by stress when people use food as a coping mechanism for unpleasant feelings or as a means to decompress. Binge eating episodes, thoughtless nibbling, and the ingestion of comfort foods that are heavy in fat, sugar, and calories might result from this. While turning to food for comfort may provide temporary relief from stress, it can also result in weight gain and make it difficult to achieve weight loss goals. Managing stress and finding healthier ways to cope can break the cycle of emotional eating and support overall well-being.

5. Erratic sleeping habits

Prolonged stress may interfere with sleep cycles and lead to poor-quality sleep, which can affect appetite control, metabolism, and weight control. Hunger hormones like ghrelin and leptin might change due to sleep loss and sleep architecture disruptions, which can increase appetite and encourage weight gain. Exhaustion and a lack of energy caused by inadequate sleep further complicate weight reduction attempts, which may lower physical activity levels and willingness to participate in healthy habits.

6. Coping Mechanisms and Stress Reduction

Efficient stress management is crucial for maintaining mental and physical health, and using constructive coping mechanisms may lessen the detrimental impact of stress on weight control. The following are some effective methods for managing stress:

Mindfulness and Meditation: Using mindfulness and meditation practices may ease anxiety, encourage calmness, and enhance emotional health. Meditation aims to quiet the mind and develop inner peace, while mindfulness focuses on being aware of the current moment without passing judgment. Frequent mindfulness and meditation practice may improve stress resilience, control hunger, and reduce cortisol levels.

Physical Activity: Being physically active daily helps lower stress levels, elevate mood, and enhance general health. Exercise helps lower cortisol levels in the body and triggers the production of endorphins, which are naturally occurring mood enhancers. Choose stress-reduction and weight-loss strategies that you love doing, such as strength training, yoga, running, or walking, and include them in your daily routine.

Healthy Lifestyle Practices: Developing healthy lifestyle practices may help lower stress and enhance general well-being. Examples of these practices include eating a balanced diet, getting enough sleep, and using relaxation methods. Make self-care activities that help you relax and relieve stress a priority. Some examples of these activities include having a warm bath, enjoying music, going outside, or pursuing interests and hobbies that make you happy.

Social Support: Retaining close social ties and asking for help from loved ones, friends, or a support group may be quite beneficial in offering emotional support when things get tough. Speaking with reliable people about your emotions and experiences may reduce stress, provide perspective, and promote a feeling of community and connection. When you need assistance, look for resources and surround yourself with supportive people.

7. Psychological Elements

Apart from the physiological consequences of stress on weight gain, psychological elements like worry, despair, and poor self-worth may also impact eating habits and lead to weight gain. People may use food as a coping mechanism for unpleasant feelings or a technique to dull emotional discomfort, leading to emotional eating and weight gain. By addressing underlying psychological problems, therapy, counseling, or support groups may assist people in improving their relationship with food and body image, as well as helping them establish better-coping skills.

8. Environmental Elements

Environmental variables that might affect weight gain and obesity rates include stress at work, socioeconomic position, the availability of healthy food alternatives, and social determinants of health. Effective stress management and the adoption of healthy lifestyle practices may provide significant challenges for those who experience socioeconomic inequalities or live in high-stress circumstances. Reducing gaps in weight-related outcomes and improving general health outcomes for all people may be achieved by addressing structural inequalities and boosting access to resources, including reasonably priced, healthy food, secure recreational areas, and mental health services.

9. Gender Differences

According to research, women are more likely than men to suffer stress-induced weight gain and emotional eating habits. This shows that there may be gender variations in the association between stress and weight gain. These gender disparities may be caused by biological, hormonal, and social variables, such as variations in body composition, cortisol metabolism, and cultural expectations around weight and body image. To manage stress-related weight gain in both men and women, customized treatments and support measures may be informed by an understanding of these gender-specific characteristics.

In conclusion, long-term stress may significantly impact physiological and psychological aspects of health, leading to weight gain and obesity. The complicated association between stress and weight gain is influenced by several variables, including elevated cortisol levels, disturbed appetite control, emotional eating patterns, and environmental circumstances. People may address psychological problems, acquire beneficial coping mechanisms, handle stress well, create supportive surroundings, and lessen the detrimental impacts of stress on their ability to control their weight and general health.

- **Stress-Reduction Methods**

Effective stress management is crucial for maintaining physical and mental health, particularly for weight control objectives. Including stress-reduction techniques in your daily routine may help you become more resilient to stress overall, decrease cortisol levels, and cut down on emotional eating. We'll look at several stress-reduction strategies in this part that may help you lose weight and improve your general health and well-being.

1. Meditation with mindfulness

One of the most effective methods for lowering stress and increasing relaxation is mindfulness meditation. It entails paying attention to the here and now without passing judgment, which enables you to develop inner serenity and tranquility. Frequent mindfulness meditation practice has been shown to promote psychological well-being overall, reduce cortisol levels, and lessen symptoms of anxiety and depression. To engage in mindfulness meditation, choose a peaceful, comfortable area, shut your eyes, and concentrate on your breathing or a particular physical experience. Gently bring your attention back to the present, acknowledging any ideas or sensations that come to mind without passing judgment on them.

2. Deep breathing exercises

Exercises that include deep breathing are simple to do yet very beneficial for lowering tension and encouraging calm. By eliciting the parasympathetic nervous system and inducing the body's relaxation response, deep breathing reduces cortisol levels. To begin practicing deep breathing, choose a peaceful, cozy spot to sit or lie down. Close your eyes and take a deep breath through your nose, allowing your abdomen to expand fully. After holding your breath for a little while, release all tension and stress with each calm, full breath out of your lips. Continue doing this for a few minutes, paying close attention to your breathing and permitting yourself to unwind completely.

3. Gradual Relaxation of the Muscles

To relieve stress and encourage relaxation, progressive muscle relaxation is a method that involves tensing and then releasing various bodily muscle groups. This method lessens tense muscles, improves body awareness, and eases symptoms of stress, including headaches, pains in the muscles, and exhaustion. To engage in progressive muscle relaxation, choose a peaceful, comfortable area where you can sit or lie down comfortably. Tense the muscles in one area of your body, starting with your toes, for a brief period. Then, release the tension and let the muscles relax fully. Make your way up to your head and neck by gradually moving through each muscle group in your body. Let go of any residual tension or stress and concentrate on the feeling of relaxation.

4. Stretching and Yoga

Stretching and yoga are mild but powerful methods for boosting relaxation, increasing flexibility, and lowering stress. Yoga creates a comprehensive strategy for reducing stress and promoting well-being by combining physical postures, breathing exercises, and meditation. Regular yoga practice has been shown to enhance the general quality of life, reduce cortisol levels, and lessen symptoms of sadness and anxiety. Whether you want a more vigorous vinyasa flow or a more calm hatha yoga practice, including yoga in your routine may assist your weight reduction goals and help manage stress. Simple stretching techniques may also aid in releasing muscular tension and stiffness, encouraging relaxation, and lowering stress levels.

5. Assisted Vision and Imagery

Using mental images to induce calm and relaxation is the goal of guided imagery and visualization treatments. Imagine serene and calm environments to induce a relaxation response in the body and lower stress levels. Audio recordings or the assistance of a qualified therapist may be used. Find a spot to sit or lie down that is quiet and comfortable. Close your eyes and picture yourself in a calm and tranquil place, such as a beach, forest, or alpine meadow. Allow yourself to let go of any tension or worry, close your eyes, and concentrate on the sights, sounds, and feelings of your imagined surroundings.

6. Keeping a Journal and Writing Expressively

Expressive writing and journaling are useful techniques for managing your emotions, lowering your stress level, and understanding your ideas and feelings. You may relieve pent-up tension, make sense of confusing ideas, and get perspective on difficult events by writing down your thoughts and feelings in a notebook or diary. Writing in a diary may be a therapeutic and uplifting activity, whether you decide to write openly about your day, make lists of your blessings, or examine certain concerns and how they affect your life. Make time every day to write in your diary and permit yourself to express yourself honestly, without fear of criticism or embarrassment.

7. Outdoor Activities and Nature

There are several advantages to being outside and spending time in nature when it comes to lowering stress and fostering calm. The body and mind are calmed by nature, which also helps reduce cortisol levels and elevate mood. Spending time in nature, whether it be via hiking, gardening, birding, or just relaxing in a peaceful park, may help you feel refreshed and less stressed. Schedule regular time to spend in nature, even if it's just for a quick stroll or a few minutes of outdoor meditation

8. Social Links and Support

Preserving close social ties and asking friends, relatives, or a support group for assistance may provide important emotional support when things are stressful. Speaking with reliable people about your emotions and experiences may reduce stress, provide perspective, and promote a feeling of community and connection. When you need assistance, look for resources and surround yourself with supportive people. Whether it's via online forums, community groups, or mealtime gatherings with loved ones, place a high value on social interaction and rely on your support system when things get tough.

9. Good living habits

Apart from using targeted methods to alleviate stress, embracing salubrious lifestyle choices may foster stress tolerance and promote general welfare. Prioritizing sleep, eating a balanced diet, exercising often, abstaining from excessive alcohol and caffeine, and managing stress may all help to improve one's physical and mental well-being. Give yourself the attention you deserve and give top priority to things that feed your body, mind, and soul. Maintaining a healthy balance in your life and managing stress more effectively may be achieved through comprehensive self-care.

- **Practices of Mindfulness**

The practice of mindfulness involves paying close attention to the current moment without passing judgment. People who practice mindfulness may become more aware of their thoughts, emotions, and sensations, which can lower stress, increase emotional control, and improve their general wellbeing. This section will discuss several mindfulness techniques and how they could help with stress reduction and weight loss.

1. Conscious breathing

Mindful breathing is among the easiest and most accessible mindfulness techniques. This is concentrating on the feelings that your breath makes as it enters and exits your body. Close your eyes and choose a comfortable sitting posture to begin practicing mindful breathing. Without attempting to alter it, start observing your breath and note your chest's rise and fall, as well as the feeling of air going through your nostrils. If your thoughts stray, bring your focus back to your breathing, softly and without passing judgment. Even a short daily practice of mindful breathing may help induce relaxation, lower stress levels, and mental calmness.

2. Meditation Using Your Body Scan

Body scan meditation is a technique that includes developing awareness of bodily sensations while methodically focusing attention on various body parts, from head to toe. This technique may reduce tension, encourage relaxation, and help people become more aware of their bodies. Close your eyes and choose a comfortable resting posture to begin a body scan meditation. Starting from your toes, progressively raise your awareness to each section of your body. As you go, note any feelings or tense spots. Give yourself permission to completely feel every emotion, free from criticism or the desire to alter anything. People may build a feeling of comfort and calm and become more conscious of their physical condition by methodically examining their bodies in this manner.

3. Conscientious consumption

The practice of mindful eating entails paying attention to all aspects of the eating experience, such as the food's flavor, texture, and sensations, as well as any thoughts or feelings that may surface. By engaging in mindful eating practices, people may foster more balanced eating habits, reduce emotional eating, and have a better connection with food.

Before meals, spend a few minutes to focus yourself and engage in mindful eating. Note your meal's appearance, smell, and hunger or fullness. Savor every mouthful of your meal and concentrate on its tastes, textures, and mouthfeel while you eat. Allow yourself to really experience the act of eating in the here and now, and notice any ideas or feelings that come up without passing judgment. People may develop a better feeling of contentment and pleasure from their food by practicing mindful mindfulness during meals, which can result in more balanced eating habits and better digestion.

4. Move with awareness.

Body, breath, and mind motions are all mindfully observed in mindful movement techniques, including yoga, tai chi, and qigong. These exercises may lower stress and improve general well-being, in addition to helping people become more flexible, relaxed, and aware of their bodies. Whether it's yoga, tai chi, or just strolling around the park, select a physical activity or exercise that you like to engage in mindful movement. As you move your body, pay attention to your breathing pattern, movement sensations, and any arising feelings or ideas. Allow yourself to move with grace and fluidity, paying attention to any regions of your body that seem tense or resistant. People may improve their physical and mental health, lessen stress, and foster a stronger feeling of vitality and energy by practicing mindful awareness while moving.

5. Meditation on kindness and love

The practice of loving-kindness meditation focuses on cultivating feelings of love, compassion, and kindness toward oneself and others. This technique may lessen stress and foster healthy connections while also assisting people in gaining more emotional well-being, empathy, and resilience. Close your eyes and choose a comfortable sitting posture to begin practicing loving-kindness meditation. Start by thinking about someone you love and care for, such as a friend, mentor, or loved one. Ask this person quietly, "May you be happy, healthy, safe, and at ease." Keep repeating these loving-kindness wishes for yourself, neutral people, and even people you may find difficult to get along with. People may improve their relationships, lessen stress, and become more emotionally resilient by practicing love and compassion for themselves and other people.

6. Everyday Mindfulness

People may develop mindfulness in their daily lives by adding attentive awareness to their routines and activities in addition to engaging in formal mindfulness practices. Basic activities like walking, brushing your teeth, and doing the dishes may be included in this. By paying close attention to the present moment, people may lower stress levels, boost happiness, and encourage a stronger sense of presence and participation in their lives. To cultivate mindfulness in your daily life, choose one or two tasks that you do often and dedicate a short period of time each day to practicing attentive awareness of them. As you participate in these activities, pay attention to the feelings, ideas, and sensations that surface and give yourself permission to be totally present. People may improve their general well-being, help them lose weight, and become more resilient to stress by practicing mindfulness in their daily lives.

Chapter 6

Sleep Well to Lose Weight

- **The Relationship Between Weight and Sleep**

Sleep is essential for controlling a wide range of physiological functions in the body, such as energy balance, metabolism, and hunger control. A disturbed sleep schedule has been connected to weight gain, obesity, and metabolic dysfunction. Make sure to get enough rest as it is essential for your overall health and happiness. This section will examine the intricate relationship between weight and sleep, including the physiological processes at play, the effects of sleep deprivation on hunger and metabolism, and doable methods for enhancing sleep to assist with weight control.

1. Control of Hormones

Many hormones that control hunger, appetite, and energy expenditure are produced and released in response to sleep. The two main hormones in this process are ghrelin and leptin. The hormone leptin, which is generated by fat cells, tells the brain when an individual is satisfied and controls energy levels. In contrast, the stomach secretes the hormone ghrelin, which increases food intake and piques hunger. It has been shown that sleep loss upsets the hormones' delicate balance, increasing the hunger-stimulating hormone ghrelin and decreasing the fullness-signaling hormone leptin. Hormonal imbalances may lead to overeating, cravings for high-calorie meals, and increased hunger, all of which can contribute to obesity and weight gain.

2. Dysregulation of Metabolism

In addition to hormonal changes, sleep deprivation may affect energy metabolism and metabolic function. Research has shown that a lack of sleep is linked to changes in insulin sensitivity, lipid metabolism, and glucose metabolism. These changes may raise the risk of obesity, type 2 diabetes, and cardiovascular disease. Prolonged sleep deprivation has been associated with increased levels of free fatty acids in the blood, insulin resistance, and poor glucose tolerance—all of which may lead to metabolic dysfunction and weight gain. Moreover, it has been shown that insufficient sleep throws off the body's circadian cycle, resulting in hormone dysregulation related to hunger, changes in energy expenditure, and a rise in fat accumulation.

3. Factors related to behavior

In addition to physiological changes, sleep deprivation may affect behavior and lifestyle variables that lead to weight gain. People who lack sleep may feel more tired, less motivated to exercise, and have trouble making decisions. These symptoms may all contribute to a reduction in physical activity and an increase in sedentary behavior. In addition, people who sleep-deprived people consume more high-calorie, high-fat meals because they are looking for rapid energy fixes to help them feel less worn out and sleepy. Lack of sleep may also affect one's ability to think clearly and exercise self-control, which makes it harder to avoid cravings and choose healthy foods.

4. Sleep duration and quality

The length and quality of sleep play a significant role in influencing how well one manages their weight. Although the ideal amount of sleep varies based on personal requirements, most individuals need seven to nine hours of sleep per night to maintain excellent health and well-being. But quality sleep is equally as important as quantity when it comes to health. Frequent awakenings, disruptions in sleep architecture, or sleep disorders like insomnia or sleep apnea are signs of poor sleep quality, which may worsen the detrimental effects of sleep on metabolism, food control, and weight management.

5. Realistic Techniques for Improving Sleep

Improving the length and quality of sleep is crucial for promoting both general health and weight control. The following are some doable methods for enhancing excellent sleep hygiene and encouraging deep, restful sleep:
Create a Regular Sleep Schedule: To help your body's internal clock and encourage a regular sleep-wake cycle, go to bed and get up at the same time every day, even on weekends.
Establish a Calm Bedtime Routine: To let your body know when it's time to wind down and get ready for sleep, establish a calm bedtime routine. This might include doing things like

reading a book, taking a warm bath, or practicing relaxation methods.

Establish a Comfortable Sleep Environment: Make sure your bedroom is quiet, dark, and cold to promote restful sleep. To reduce noise, choose a comfortable mattress and pillows, and think about using earplugs, white noise machines, or blackout curtains.

Minimize Stimulants and Electronics Before Bed: Alcohol, nicotine, and caffeine should not be consumed just before bed since they might disrupt your sleep. Limit your exposure to screens and electronic devices, such as TVs, laptops, and cell phones. The blue light these gadgets generate might interfere with the body's natural synthesis of melatonin, a hormone that controls sleep and waking cycles.

Practice Relaxation Techniques: To relieve tension and encourage relaxation before bed, try deep breathing, meditation, or progressive muscle relaxation.

Limit Daytime Naps: Although brief naps during the day may be helpful for some people, taking too many naps during the day might interfere with sleep at night and throw off the sleep-wake cycle. If you must snooze, try to get in a quick 20–30-minute sleep in the early afternoon.

Exercise frequently: Participate in regular physical activity throughout the day, which may improve the quality and quantity of your sleep. But steer clear of strenuous activity just before bed, as it may impede the start of sleep.

- **Creating a Restful Sleep Schedule**

To promote deep, rejuvenating sleep and preserve general health and well-being, it is important to follow a healthy sleep pattern, also referred to as sleep hygiene. You can maximize the quality of your sleep and awaken each morning feeling rejuvenated by forming regular sleep routines and setting up a sleep-friendly atmosphere. This section will include helpful hints and techniques for creating a regular sleep schedule that encourages deep, rejuvenating sleep.

1. Establish a regular sleep schedule.

Keeping a regular sleep schedule is one of the most crucial components of a healthy sleep pattern. To maintain a healthy sleep-wake cycle and regulate your body's internal clock, try to go to bed and get up at the same time every day, even on weekends. To help your body create a regular rhythm and maximize the quality of your sleep, consistency is essential.

2. Establish a calm nighttime routine.

Developing a calming evening routine can effectively signal to your body that it's time to relax and prepare for sleep. Take up soothing hobbies like reading a book, taking a warm bath, or practicing relaxation methods like deep breathing or meditation. Avoid stimulating activities before bed, such as watching TV or using electronics, because the blue light they produce may interfere with the generation of melatonin and make it difficult for you to fall asleep.

3. Improve your sleeping environment.

Establish a relaxing tranquil, sleep-inducing atmosphere in your home. To reduce noise, make sure your bedroom is cold, quiet, and dark. You may also want to use earplugs, white noise generators, or blackout curtains. Purchase pillows and a comfy mattress that will support your body well. Eliminate any light or noise sources that can keep you awake at night.

4. Before sleeping, limit electronics and stimulants.

When it comes to going to bed, stay away from stimulants like coffee, nicotine, and alcohol since these may make it difficult for you to fall asleep and ruin your sleep. In the hour before bed, limit your time spent in front of displays and electronic devices, including computers, TVs, and cell phones. These gadgets' blue light may interfere with your circadian clock and reduce melatonin synthesis, making it more difficult to fall asleep.

5. Utilize calming methods.

To help you relax before bed and to help quiet your body and mind, include relaxation exercises in your evening routine. Progressive muscle relaxation, guided visualization, and deep breathing exercises are all useful methods for lowering tension and anxiety and encouraging sound sleep. Try different relaxation methods to find your favorite, then incorporate them into your daily routine.

6. Limit Your Daytime Napping

While short naps during the day may be helpful for some people, taking too many naps throughout the day might interfere with your ability to fall asleep at night and throw off your sleep-wake cycle. If you must take a nap during the day, try to schedule a quick 20–30-minute nap in the early afternoon to prevent disrupting your sleep at night. Refrain from taking naps too close to bedtime, as this might interfere with your ability to fall asleep at night.

7. Participate in regular exercise.

Frequent physical exercise during the day may improve sleep quality and encourage peaceful slumber. Try to avoid doing intense activity too soon before bedtime, as it may excite your body and make it more difficult to fall asleep. Instead, aim for at least 30 minutes of moderate-to-intense exercise most days of the week. Include enjoyable physical activities in your daily routine, such as cycling, swimming, running, or walking.

8. Control your anxiety and stress.

The inability to fall and remain asleep may be caused by stress and worry; therefore, it's important to learn good coping mechanisms and relaxation techniques. Incorporate relaxation exercises into your routine and practice stress-reduction methods, including progressive muscle relaxation, deep breathing, and meditation. To help you better manage stress and anxiety, you should also make an effort to address the causes of stress in your life and create coping mechanisms.

9. Examine your sleep environment.

Examine your sleeping environment carefully and adapt as needed to maximize your sleep quality. Take into account elements like the comfort of your pillows and mattress, the lighting and temperature in your bedroom, and any potential sources of noise or disruption that could be affecting your ability to sleep. Make the necessary adjustments to create a sleeping environment that promotes deep, rejuvenating sleep.

10. If needed, seek professional assistance.

If you've tried a variety of methods to create a healthy sleep schedule but are still having trouble falling asleep, you may want to consult a doctor or sleep expert for assistance. They may assist in identifying any underlying medical issues or sleep disorders that may be interfering with your ability to sleep, as well as suggesting suitable therapies or treatments to support you in obtaining the necessary quality sleep.

Chapter 7

Altering Your Lifestyle for Long-Term Weight Loss

- **Including Movement in Your Daily Routine**

A healthy lifestyle must include physical exercise, which is also essential for long-term weight reduction. You may increase your energy expenditure, strengthen and extend your endurance, improve your cardiovascular health, and improve your general well-being by moving throughout the day. In this section, we'll look at doable methods for adding exercise to your daily schedule to help you reach your weight reduction goals and encourage an active lifestyle.

1. Establish sensible objectives.

Setting attainable objectives that meet your tastes, lifestyle, and current level of fitness is crucial when adding exercise to your day. Begin by determining what you enjoy doing and how it fits into your schedule. Examples of such activities include dance, swimming, walking, running, cycling, and group fitness courses. Establish quantifiable, precise objectives for the frequency and length of your weekly physical exercise, and gradually increase the intensity and duration as your strength and endurance improve.

2. Look for chances to relocate.

Seek chances to move more throughout your everyday schedule, both at work and at home. To save steps, park farther away from your destination, walk or ride your bike to neighboring errands, or use the stairs instead of the elevator. Every hour, stretch or take little walks to break up extended periods of sitting. To remind yourself to get up and exercise throughout the day, set up alerts on your phone or calendar.

3. Plan frequent exercise times.

Plan regular workout sessions into your weekly calendar in addition to impromptu activities throughout the day. Aim for 75 minutes of vigorous-intensity aerobic exercise or at least 150 minutes of moderate-intensity aerobic activity each week, in addition to two or more days of muscle-strengthening activities. Whether it's running, working out at the gym, or lifting weights, choose pursuits that you love and that provide a physical challenge.

4. Make exercise fun.

By selecting things that you love and look forward to, you may turn physical exercise into a pleasurable and entertaining part of your day. Try a variety of exercises to see what suits you the best: sports, dance, hiking, yoga, or other physical activities. To help the time fly quickly, invite friends or family to join you for exercises or outdoor activities. You may also listen to music or podcasts while working out.

5. Allocate a specific time for exercise.

Make physical activity a priority by dedicating a specific amount of time each day to exercise. Put exercise on your calendar like any other important event. Whether it's first thing in the morning, during your lunch break, or in the evening after work, decide when you feel most energized and inspired to work out. Consistency is required to develop a regular workout program and make physical activity an essential part of your daily routine.

6. Change up your daily schedule.

A variety of exercises and activities may be added to your fitness program to keep things fresh and avoid monotony. Consider taking up new fitness courses, going on adventures on various outdoor paths or trails, or setting new fitness goals for yourself. Combining aerobic, strength, flexibility, and balance exercises with cross-training may help reduce the risk of overuse injuries, enhance general fitness, and keep you motivated and interested in your workouts.

7. Pay attention to your body.

During exercise, pay attention to your body's signals and pay heed to any signs of exhaustion, pain, or discomfort. In order to achieve your objectives and push yourself to the maximum, remember when to take breaks and recuperate to avoid burnout and injuries. Include rest days in your weekly schedule to give your body the time it needs to heal and rebuild, and give special attention to activities that help you decompress and relieve tension, like yoga, meditation, or light stretching.

8. Stay steady and relentless.

Maintaining a healthy lifestyle and attaining lasting weight reduction require perseverance and consistency. Even on the days when you don't feel inspired or motivated, stick to your fitness regimen and prioritize being outside. Recall that little, gradual changes accumulate over time, and that progress is a slow process. Celebrate your victories and accomplishments along the way, and don't let difficulties or disappointments deter you. Continue taking one step at a time and keep your eyes on your long-term objectives.

- **Ways to Keep Moving Even When Not Doing Traditional Exercise**

Maintaining general health and well-being requires regular physical activity, which doesn't have to include rigorous exercises or scheduled gym visits. Without partaking in conventional exercise, there are many other methods to maintain your level of activity and add movement to your daily schedule. This section will discuss doable methods for maintaining an active lifestyle throughout the day, both at home and at work, in order to help you reach your weight reduction objectives.

1. Incorporate more movement into your daily work.

Seek chances to move more throughout your regular jobs and hobbies. Try to add additional steps to your day by using the stairs whenever you can, rather than utilizing contemporary conveniences like escalators and elevators. When watching TV or chatting on the phone, get up and walk around. You may also utilize the commercial breaks to do brief stretches or exercises. Short walks or domestic duties like cleaning, vacuuming, or gardening might help break up extended periods of sitting.

2. Make active transportation decisions.

To add extra activity to your everyday routine, wherever feasible, opt for active modes of transportation. Rather than driving, choose to walk or ride a bike to your destination, or use public transit and walk to and from the stops and stations. If you must drive, park farther away from your destination to accrue more steps; alternatively, for quick errands, think about bicycling or walking. You'll not only increase your physical activity level but also lower your carbon footprint and save money on gasoline.

3. Participate in recreational activities and hobbies.

To appreciate being active, look for pastimes and leisure pursuits that require movement and physical exertion. Think of enjoyable and lifestyle-fitting hobbies such as hiking, bicycling, swimming, dancing, gardening, or sports. Discover new outdoor leisure possibilities and activities by exploring your local parks, trails, or recreational facilities. To increase the enjoyment and satisfaction of your social gatherings and physical trips, ask friends or family to join you.

4. Incorporate exercise into your social and family activities.

During family and social events, prioritize being active by selecting activities that require mobility and physical exertion. Suggest taking a walk or hike together, playing outdoor activities like volleyball or frisbee, or signing up for group fitness classes or sports leagues as an alternative to getting together for lunch or coffee. Arrange physically demanding activities or excursions for yourself and your loved ones. Some ideas include going to an aquarium or zoo, strolling around a new neighborhood or city, or spending a day at a local nature reserve or theme park.

5. Utilize technology to remain engaged.

To maintain your motivation and level of activity throughout the day, use technology to your advantage. To keep track of your daily steps, activity levels, and physical activity objectives, use fitness trackers or smartphone applications. Participate in virtual fitness challenges or events by connecting with others who share your interests and ambitions by joining online communities or social media groups dedicated to fitness. Use fitness apps to get individualized exercise regimens and training plans, or watch workout videos or take online exercise courses for direction and inspiration.

6. Increase the activity level of daily activities.

Seek methods to add activity and challenge to routine tasks to boost energy expenditure and encourage muscular activation. While you're waiting for things to boil or cook, stand up and do simple exercises like calf raises, lunges, or squats instead of sitting down to read or watch TV. For strength training activities, use common household objects like cans or water bottles as improvised weights. You can also incorporate balancing exercises, such as standing on one leg while doing the dishes or brushing your teeth.

7. Make small, doable goals.

To increase the amount of activity in your everyday routine, set modest, attainable objectives and acknowledge your accomplishments as you go. To begin, make a goal to walk 10,000 steps a day or to do moderate-to-intense physical activity for at least half of the days of the week. As you gain strength and endurance, gradually increase the amount of exercise you do. You should also push yourself to try new things and work out longer or harder. No matter how little, acknowledge and celebrate your accomplishments and milestones, and use them as fuel to keep advancing toward your objectives.

Creating a Healthy Environment for Weight Loss

A healthy environment is essential for promoting weight reduction because it offers the structures, tools, and support needed to encourage healthy choices and behaviors. In order to assist your weight reduction objectives, we'll look at doable tactics in this part for setting up a healthy atmosphere that encourages a balanced diet, frequent exercise, and general well-being.

1. Store nutritious foods in your kitchen.

Begin by arranging a range of wholesome items in your kitchen that will aid in your weight-reduction efforts. Keep whole, minimally processed foods like fruits, veggies, whole grains, lean meats, and healthy fats in your pantry, fridge, and freezer. Store wholesome snacks nearby for when you become hungry, and try to avoid having too many highly processed, high-calorie items around to entice you to overindulge.

2. Arrange and cook nutritious meals.

To make sure you always have wholesome alternatives accessible throughout the week, take the effort to plan and prepare healthy meals in advance. Set aside time every week to shop for supplies, create a shopping list, and plan your meals. To prepare nutritious meals and snacks ahead of time that can be quickly assembled or reheated during hectic weekdays, think about batch cooking or meal preparation on the weekends. To encourage fullness and avoid overeating, concentrate on including a balance of protein, fiber, and healthy fats in each meal.

3. Establish a helpful social network.

Embrace a social network of friends, family, or peers who are as committed to your health and fitness as you are. Find people who can hold you accountable, inspire you to make healthy choices, and support you in your attempts. Joining a support group, exercise class, or online community may help you connect with others going through a similar experience and exchange advice, information, and encouragement.

4. Make exercise accessible and convenient.

By eliminating any hurdles and difficulties that could prevent you from exercising, you can include physical activity into your daily routine in a comfortable and accessible way. Pick enjoyable activities that you can incorporate into your schedule, such as cycling, swimming, walking, running, or group fitness sessions. Look for opportunities to walk or bike to local locations, park farther away from your destination to get in additional steps, or use the stairs rather than the elevator as a way to incorporate movement into your everyday routines.

5. Create a successful environment.

Create a conducive atmosphere for achievement by choosing healthily when it's convenient. Make sure your exercise gear and attire are always accessible and visible to act as a reminder to work out on a regular basis. Make specific areas of your house for physical activity, like a home gym or workout room, and fill them with fun-to-use training gear and accessories. Make sure that bad meals are kept out of sight and replaced with healthier options to reduce signals and triggers that may encourage unhealthy behavior.

6. Eat mindfully and control your portion sizes.

To encourage healthy eating habits and avoid overindulging, practice portion management and mindful eating. Eat slowly and deliberately to appreciate the tastes and textures of your meal, and pay attention to your body's signals of hunger and fullness. To help manage portion sizes, use smaller dishes, plates, and utensils. Eating straight out of packages or containers might result in thoughtless overindulgence. To prevent overindulging and distracted eating, practice portion control by measuring and portioning out your food ahead of time. You may also avoid eating in front of a computer or TV.

7. Establish a calm and peaceful atmosphere.

To improve your general health and well-being, learn to manage stress and establish a calming atmosphere. To induce relaxation and lower stress levels, try stress-reduction methods like yoga, meditation, or deep breathing. Make sleep a priority by providing a comfortable sleeping environment that promotes peaceful, restorative sleep. Create a relaxing nighttime ritual to help you relax and prepare for sleep. Make self-care activities that help you relax and relieve stress a priority. Some examples of these activities include reading a book, taking a bath, or going for a walk outdoors.

8. Keep track of your progress and make any necessary changes.

Track your progress toward your weight reduction objectives and, if necessary, modify your surroundings and habits to remain on course. Using a notebook, app, or monitoring tool, record your food consumption, exercise, and weight loss progress. Then, periodically evaluate your results to see trends, patterns, and areas that might need improvement. To overcome any difficulties or problems that may arise along the way, be adaptable and ready to make adjustments to your habits and surroundings as necessary.

Keep in mind that making small adjustments over time can have a significant impact, and maintaining your weight loss goals necessitates creating a healthy environment.

Summary

Adopting a Well-Being Lifestyle for Durable Outcomes

In the process of reaching and keeping a healthy weight, it's critical to understand that long-term benefits come from adopting a balanced lifestyle that places an emphasis on wholesome food, consistent exercise, and general wellbeing rather than from quick fixes or fad diets. Achieving long-lasting benefits that improve your health and quality of life may be facilitated by implementing sustainable habits and beneficial adjustments to your surroundings, behaviors, and mentality.

Maintaining a Healthy Diet and Exercise Schedule

The requirements for a balanced lifestyle begin with a diet rich in nutrients and regular exercise. Make an effort to eat a range of whole, minimally processed meals that fuel your body and provide vital nutrients for optimum well-being. Limit your consumption of processed meals, sugary snacks, and high-calorie drinks. Instead, include a variety of fruits, vegetables, whole grains, lean proteins, and healthy fats in your diet. Combine a healthy diet with frequent exercise to promote weight reduction, increase fitness, and improve general well being.

Setting Your Own Health and Well-Being First

Prioritizing self-care and well-being is crucial as part of a balanced lifestyle, in addition to proper diet and exercise. Make time for rest and relaxation, stress management, and rejuvenation-promoting activities. Engage in deep breathing techniques, mindfulness, or meditation to boost emotional resilience and mental clarity while lowering stress. Prioritize your sleep by developing a regular sleep schedule and a sleep-friendly atmosphere that encourages deep, rejuvenating slumber.

Establishing a helpful environment

For long-term success to be sustained, an atmosphere that is encouraging and supports healthy choices and behaviors must be established. Embrace a social network of friends, family, or peers who are supportive of your fitness and health goals and can provide accountability, inspiration, and support as you go. Organize your workspace and home to support success by keeping a well-stocked kitchen, facilitating simple access to physical exercise, and designing areas that encourage unwinding and stress reduction.

Honoring Development and Preserving Energy

It's important to recognize your achievements and celebrate your successes as you adopt a balanced lifestyle and make healthy adjustments to support your weight reduction goals. Celebrate not just the number on the scale but also the non-scale successes, such as greater energy levels, increased strength and endurance, and enhanced general well-being. Continue to put your health and fitness first, set new objectives, and push yourself to do new things, and you'll stay inspired and keep up the momentum.

Accepting the journey

Recall that attaining long-lasting outcomes is a journey that calls for constant focus, effort, and commitment rather than a destination. Accept the path towards a better, healthier version of yourself and acknowledge that obstacles and failures are normal parts of the process. When embarking on a weight reduction journey, have an optimistic outlook, be patient, and concentrate on making long-lasting changes that will benefit your overall health and wellbeing. Living a healthy lifestyle and prioritizing self-care can help you reap long-term benefits and have the best possible life.

Appendix

Sources of Additional Assistance

It's crucial to have access to trustworthy information, direction, and support as you start your weight reduction journey and work to maintain a healthy lifestyle. You may get helpful support and guidance from the following sites to help you reach your fitness and health objectives:

1. Certified Nutritionists and Dietitians

A qualified dietitian or nutritionist consultation may provide individualized advice and suggestions catered to your unique nutritional requirements, tastes, and objectives. These experts can guide you through the process of creating a balanced diet plan, making informed food choices, and resolving any issues or problems you may be having with nutrition.

2. Fitness instructors and certified personal trainers

You may get professional advice and assistance in creating a successful workout regimen, setting reasonable fitness objectives, and maintaining motivation and accountability for your fitness program by working with a certified personal trainer or fitness coach. These experts can provide you with encouragement, technique guidance, and individualized workout routines to help you reach your fitness goals in a safe and efficient manner.

3. Virtual Communities for Health and Fitness

You can meet like-minded people who share your health and fitness goals by joining online forums or support groups. These people can provide you with encouragement, inspiration, and support as you strive toward your goals. In addition to providing excellent tools, pointers, and advice on health in general, exercise, and nutrition, these communities often provide opportunities for social interaction via forums, social media groups, and online gatherings.

4. Websites and Apps for Wellbeing

Numerous websites and applications dedicated to wellness are accessible, providing a wealth of information, programs, and resources to help you on your path to better health and fitness. These tools may assist you in assessing your progress, setting goals, managing your food intake and physical activity, and accessing educational materials and support from the comfort of your own home. They range from meal planning and monitoring applications to fitness tracking gadgets and exercise programs.

5. Publications on Health and Fitness

Publications related to health and fitness, including books, periodicals, and websites, may provide you with inspiration, advice, and useful knowledge to help you achieve your wellness and weight reduction objectives. Seek reliable information sources that provide guidance and suggestions based on research for subjects including exercise, stress management, diet, and general well-being. You could choose to read books authored by professionals in the field, subscribe to health and fitness periodicals, or follow trustworthy blogs about wellbeing.

6. Resources for Local Health and Wellbeing

Investigate the programs, activities, and services that local health and wellness organizations in your region—such as gyms, fitness centers, community centers, and recreational centers—offer to help you achieve your fitness and health objectives. Additionally, a lot of towns have free or inexpensive services like jogging or walking clubs, group exercise classes, nutrition seminars, and wellness events that give you the chance to meet new people and get support and direction on your path to improved health.

Easy and Quick Recipes for a Busy Day

It might be difficult to find the time to cook healthy meals, particularly on hectic days when you're exhausted. To make meal preparation simpler and ensure that you can still enjoy healthy meals even when you're short on time, you need to have quick and straightforward recipes on hand. Here are a few quick and simple meals that you can prepare quickly on hectic days:

1. Vegetables and Chicken on a Sheet Pan

components: chicken thighs or breasts
A variety of veggies (carrots, broccoli, zucchini, and bell peppers) Olive oil
Paprika, onion powder, garlic powder, salt, and pepper

- Guidelines:
Remember to adjust the oven temperature to 400°F or 200°C.

2. Arrange the veggies and chicken on a large sheet pan and cut them into bite-sized pieces.
3. Add a drizzle of olive oil and season with salt, pepper, paprika, onion powder, and garlic powder.
4. Spread out in a single layer on the sheet pan after tossing everything together until it is equally covered.
5. Bake for 20 to 25 minutes, or until the veggies are soft and the chicken is cooked through.

2. Chickpea and vegetable quinoa salad

Cooked quinoa, washed and drained canned chickpeas, and a variety of veggies (such as cherry tomatoes, cucumbers, bell peppers, and red onions) are the ingredients.
Fresh herbs, like cilantro or parsley
Lemon juice
Olive oil
Pepper and salt
- Guidelines:
1. Put the cooked quinoa, chopped veggies, chickpeas, and fresh herbs in a big bowl.
2. After adding a drizzle of lemon juice and olive oil, taste and add salt and pepper as needed.
3. Mix everything together until well mixed, then serve right now or store in the fridge for later.

3. Tofu-Veggie Stir-Fry

Ingredients: dried and diced firm tofu; a variety of veggies (carrots, broccoli, snap peas, and bell peppers)
Soy sauce
Sesame oil
Minced garlic
grated ginger
Prepared noodles or rice
- Guidelines:
1. Heat a little amount of sesame oil in a big pan or wok and heat it over medium-high heat.
In the pan, add the cubed tofu and cook until it becomes golden brown on both sides.

3. After adding the grated ginger and minced garlic to the pan, cook for an additional minute.

4. Include the mixed veggies in the pan and stir-fry them until they become crisp-tender.

5. Pour soy sauce over everything and mix it well.

6. To finish the dish, serve the stir-fry over cooked rice or noodles.

4. Fruit and Nut Greek Yogurt Parfait

Components: Greek yogurt

A variety of fresh or frozen fruits, including pineapple, mango, and berries

Nuts or seeds, such as chia seeds, walnuts, or almonds

Optional: honey or maple syrup.

- Guidelines:

1. Arrange Greek yogurt, fresh or frozen fruit, and nuts or seeds in a serving dish or glass.

2. If preferred, drizzle with honey or maple syrup for extra sweetness.

3. Continue layering until the bowl or glass is full, and then serve right away for a healthy and expedient breakfast or snack.

Simple and quick dishes come in handy on hectic days when you need a healthy supper quickly. These simple and tasty recipes can help you maintain your fitness and health goals even when life gets busy, whether you're making a Greek yogurt parfait, putting together a quinoa salad, stir-frying vegetables with tofu, or preparing a sheet pan meal.